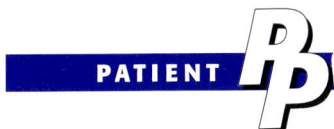

PATIENT *PP*

Clinical drawings for

Bladder disorders

by Eboo Versi MD PhD MRCOG
Associate Professor of Obstetrics,
Gynecology and Reproductive Biology,
Harvard Medical School, Boston, USA

and Timothy J Christmas MD FRCS
Consultant Urological Surgeon,
Charing Cross Hospital,
London, UK

Series Editor: J Richard Smith MD MRCOG
Consultant Gynaecologist, Chelsea and
Westminster Hospital, London, UK,
and Honorary Consultant Gynaecologist,
Royal Brompton Hospital, London, UK

Illustrated by
Dee McLean, MeDee Art, London, UK

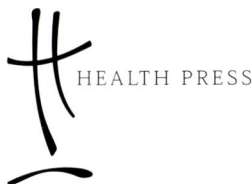

HEALTH PRESS

Oxford

Patient Pictures – Bladder disorders
First published 1998

© 1998 Health Press Limited
Elizabeth House, Queen Street,
Abingdon, Oxford, OX14 3JR, UK

A CIP catalogue record for this title is available from the
British Library.

ISBN 1-899541-37-3

Dee McLean thanks Jane Fallows for her help with
the illustrations.

Printed by Ethedo, High Wycombe, UK

Reproduction authorization

The purchaser of this *Patient Pictures* series title is hereby authorized to reproduce by photocopy only, any part of the pictorial and textual material contained in this work for non-profit, educational, or patient education use. Photocopying for these purposes only is welcomed and free from further permission requirements from the publisher and free from any fee.

The reproduction of any material from this publication outside the guidelines above is strictly prohibited without the permission in writing of the publisher and is subject to minimum charges laid down by the Publishers Licensing Society Limited or its nominees.

Sarah Redston

Publisher, Health Press Limited, Oxford

Authors' preface

As humans evolved from walking on all fours to walking on two legs, the pelvic floor, the original function of which was to allow control of micturition and defecation, had to provide gravitational support for all of the abdominal contents. Indeed, all this has to be done by a muscle that did little more than 'wag a tail' previously! This can become particularly problematic for women as the birth canal also traverses the pelvic floor. As a result, incontinence is one of the most common urological conditions, which causes significant problems for patients and their relatives.

Eboo Versi

Translating the complex language used by doctors to describe the anatomy and physiology of the lower urinary tract to patients contemplating therapy is always a problem. This book aims to try and overcome this difficulty by providing pictures and simple text that will help healthcare professionals talk through the issues in a way that patients can easily understand. The emphasis of the book is on clarity and simplicity, and so by its nature, many of the intricate details will be glossed over. The book is not intended as a comprehensive work for either the doctor or the patient, but rather as a communication tool to enhance the interaction between the two.

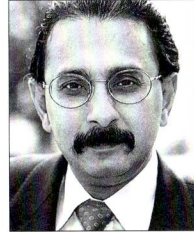

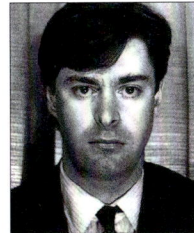

Timothy J Christmas

Eboo Versi MD PhD MRCOG
Associate Professor of Obstetrics, Gynecology and Reproductive Biology,
Harvard Medical School, Boston, USA

Timothy J Christmas MD FRCS
Consultant Urological Surgeon,
Charing Cross Hospital, London, UK

The lower urinary tract

- The bladder is like a balloon, but the wall is made of thin muscle instead of rubber. It acts as a reservoir for urine and is normally kept tightly closed by a ring of muscle called the urethral sphincter.

- The bladder gradually fills over a period of 3 – 4 hours and, when it is full, you become aware of the need to pass urine. During urination, urine passes from the bladder down the urethra to the outside. This involves relaxation of the muscles of the urethra and contraction of the bladder muscle.

- The urethra is much longer in men than in women, and the sphincter that keeps the bladder closed is also much stronger. As a result, leakage of urine is more common in women and difficulties in emptying the bladder are more common in men.

- The bladder is supported by the pelvic floor muscles. These muscles can become weakened during pregnancy and childbirth, and as a result of ageing. Part of this weakness is thought to be due to hormonal changes.

- In most women, the symptoms that occur in pregnancy disappear after the baby is born. In some women, however, the structures that support the bladder may be permanently damaged.

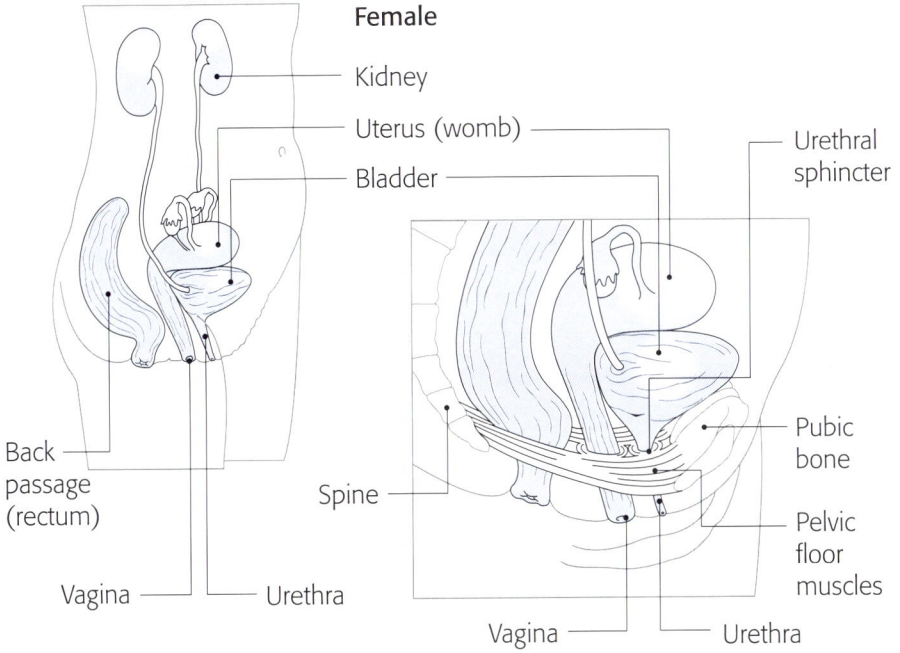

Female

Kidney

Uterus (womb)

Bladder

Urethral sphincter

Pubic bone

Back passage (rectum)

Spine

Pelvic floor muscles

Vagina

Urethra

Vagina

Urethra

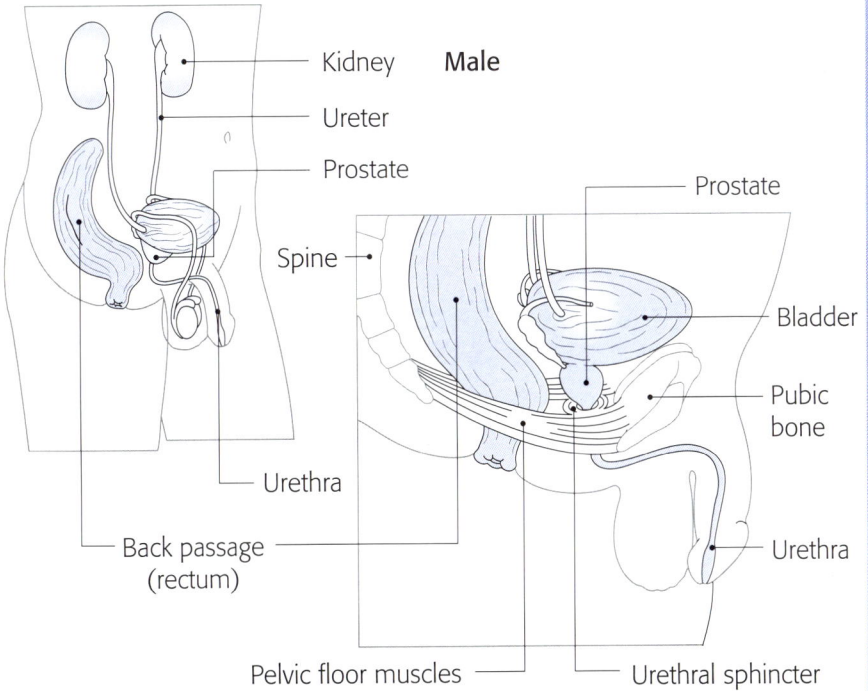

Kidney

Male

Ureter

Prostate

Spine

Prostate

Bladder

Pubic bone

Urethra

Back passage (rectum)

Urethra

Pelvic floor muscles

Urethral sphincter

Cystoscopy

- Cystoscopy is examination of the lining of the bladder using a thin 'telescope' called a cystoscope, which is passed up the urethra into the bladder. There are two types of cystoscope – flexible and rigid.

- Flexible cystoscopy is usually performed to discover the cause of a symptom, such as blood in the urine. Rigid cystoscopy allows various minor procedures to be performed at the same time, such as taking tissue samples or biopsies.

- Flexible cystoscopy is performed under a local anaesthetic. Although rigid cystoscopy can be performed under local anaesthesia, a spinal or light general anaesthetic is often preferred, particularly for men.

- Flexible cystoscopy is performed as a day-case procedure and you will be able to go home soon afterwards. Rigid cystoscopy may also be performed as a day-case, but if any other procedure, such as tissue sampling, has been performed, you may need to stay in hospital overnight.

- After the procedure, you may experience some discomfort when passing urine, but this should settle within a day or so. You will be asked to drink extra fluids for 24 hours and may be given antibiotics to help reduce the risk of infection.

- If you develop a temperature or symptoms of cystitis, you may require a full course of antibiotics and should consult your doctor.

Male

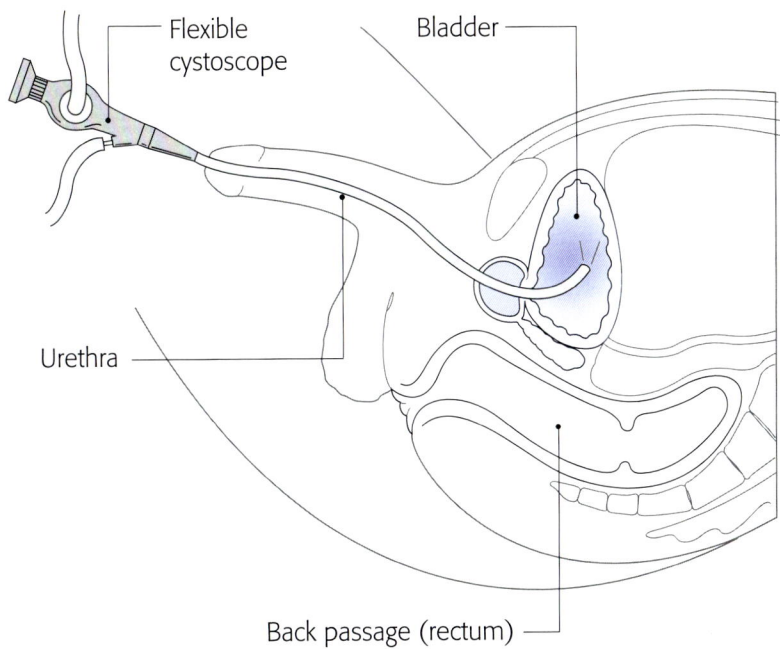

Flexible cystoscope

Bladder

Urethra

Back passage (rectum)

Female

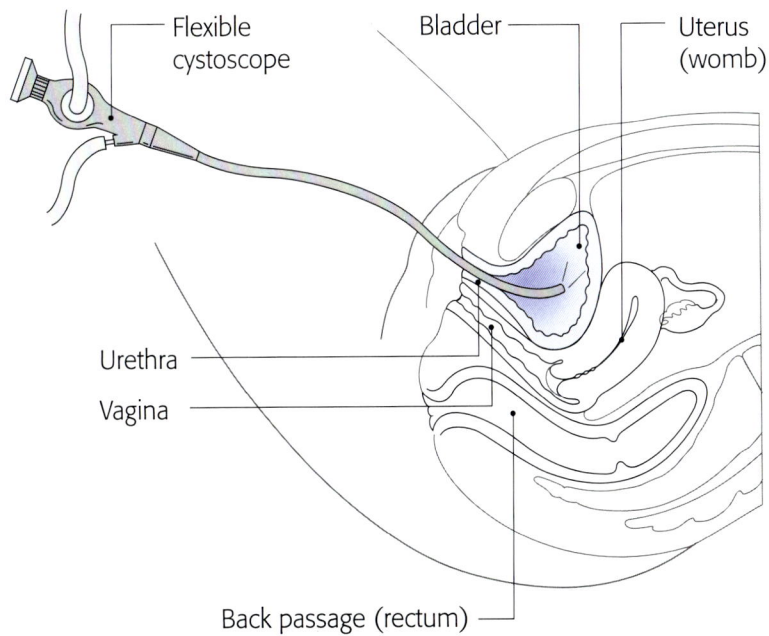

Flexible cystoscope

Bladder

Uterus (womb)

Urethra

Vagina

Back passage (rectum)

Pad testing

- A pad test is used to confirm whether the fluid that is leaking is urine, as the dampness could be due to another cause, for example, vaginal discharge.

- You may be given a pill containing pyridium, which will make your urine turn orange in colour, and you will be asked to wear a pad. When the pad becomes wet and the wet patch is coloured orange, it confirms that urine is being leaked.

- The pad weighing test may be performed to find out how much urine is being leaked. This will help to assess how severe the problem is. The test involves weighing the pad before and after it is worn, and can be carried out in the GP's surgery, doctor's office, in hospital or at home.

- Various types of pad test are carried out in hospital. These include the short pad test, the stress pad test, and the 1-hour standardized pad test. Different activities are carried out during these tests, but they all cause urine loss. For all of the tests, you will need to have a full bladder, wear the pad, and then carry out a series of exercises to stress the bladder.

- The home pad test can be either a 1-day or a 2-day test and, during this time, the patient wears as many pads as necessary. At the end of this period, all the pads are weighed together to give an idea of how much urine was lost over the 1–2 days that the pads were worn. This test is used to assess when during the day the incontinence is worse, and how well the treatment has worked.

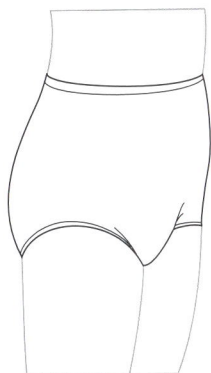

Pad

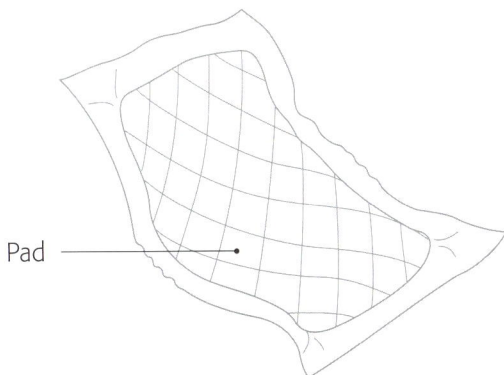

Activities carried out during pad tests

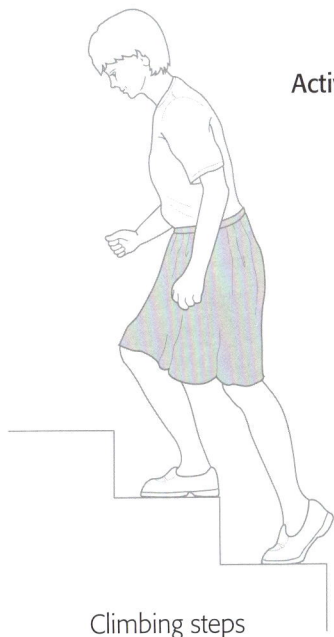

Climbing steps

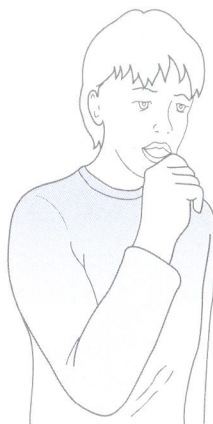

Coughing

Uroflowmetry and post-void residual volume

- Uroflowmetry is a test that measures the rate at which urine is passed. If the flow rate is slow, it is likely that either there is a blockage in the urethra or that the bladder is not contracting very well.

- You will be asked to arrive for the test with a full bladder, and to urinate into a special device called a uroflowmeter through a funnel. Ideally, this should be done in the privacy of a toilet where there is a commode.

- The uroflowmeter prints out a trace that shows how fast the urine was passed.

- Normally, the bladder is completely empty after going to the toilet. In some disorders, this does not occur. Urine that is not emptied is called the post-void residual urine.

- The post-void residual urine can be measured by either inserting a catheter up the urethra to drain the remaining urine from the bladder or by ultrasound.

- Ultrasound is a painless test in which a probe covered in a special jelly is placed on the abdomen. This enables a picture of the bladder to be taken. A computer inside the ultrasound machine is then used to calculate how much urine has been left behind in the bladder.

- Uroflowmetry and post-void residual urine measurement tests are carried out in the doctor's office or in a hospital. It takes about half an hour to complete both tests. Your doctor will often discuss the results with you straight away, and may suggest further tests or treatment.

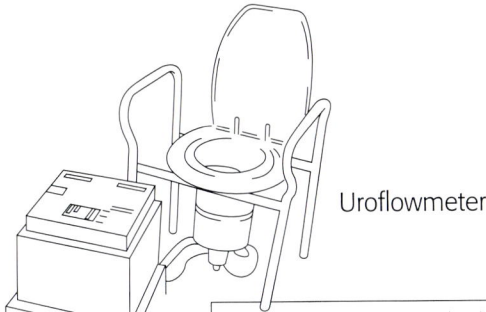

Uroflowmeter

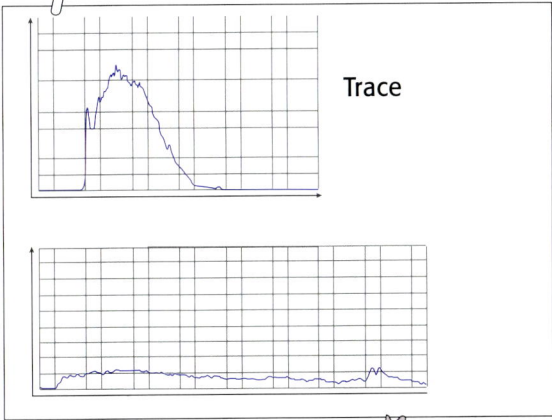

Trace

Normal urine flow

Reduced flow caused
by obstruction or
by bladder not
contracting well

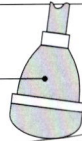

Ultrasound probe

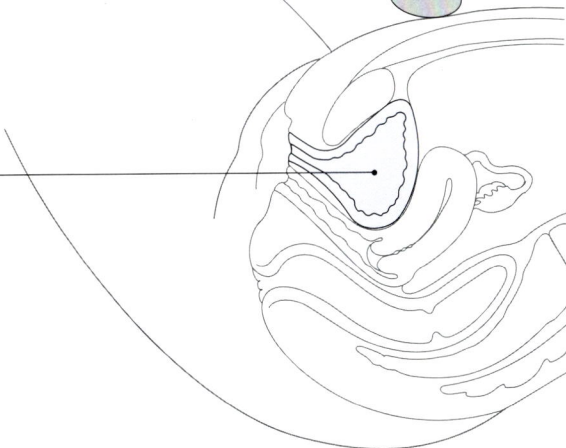

Bladder

Three-channel cystometry (urodynamics)

- Three-channel cystometry shows how the bladder is working as it fills and empties. It involves measuring three things – the pressure inside the bladder, the pressure in the abdomen and the rate at which urine is emptied from the bladder. The test takes about half an hour.

- The pressure inside the bladder may be measured using a catheter with a special sensor on the end. The pressure in the abdomen is usually measured by inserting a catheter into the back passage or rectum, though in women a vaginal catheter may be used. The bladder catheter is inserted before the rectal or vaginal catheter. To measure the flow rate, patients urinate through a funnel into a special device called a uroflowmeter.

- The bladder may be filled by drinking fluid. However, usually, it is necessary to know precisely how much fluid is in the bladder at any time. In this case, the bladder will be filled with a dilute solution of salt through the catheter.

- As the bladder is being filled, you will be asked to tell the doctor when you feel the first desire, and then a strong desire, to pass urine. After this point, the bladder will continue to be filled until you feel that you really cannot take any more. Do not be embarrassed if you leak urine during this test – the doctor expects this to happen.

- Once the bladder is completely full, you may be asked to carry out some activities, such as changing position or coughing, that could cause leakage of urine.

- You will then be asked to urinate into a uroflowmeter.

Uterus (womb)

Catheter in bladder

Catheter in vagina

Back passage (rectum)

Catheter in rectum

Catheter in bladder

Uroflowmeter

Trace

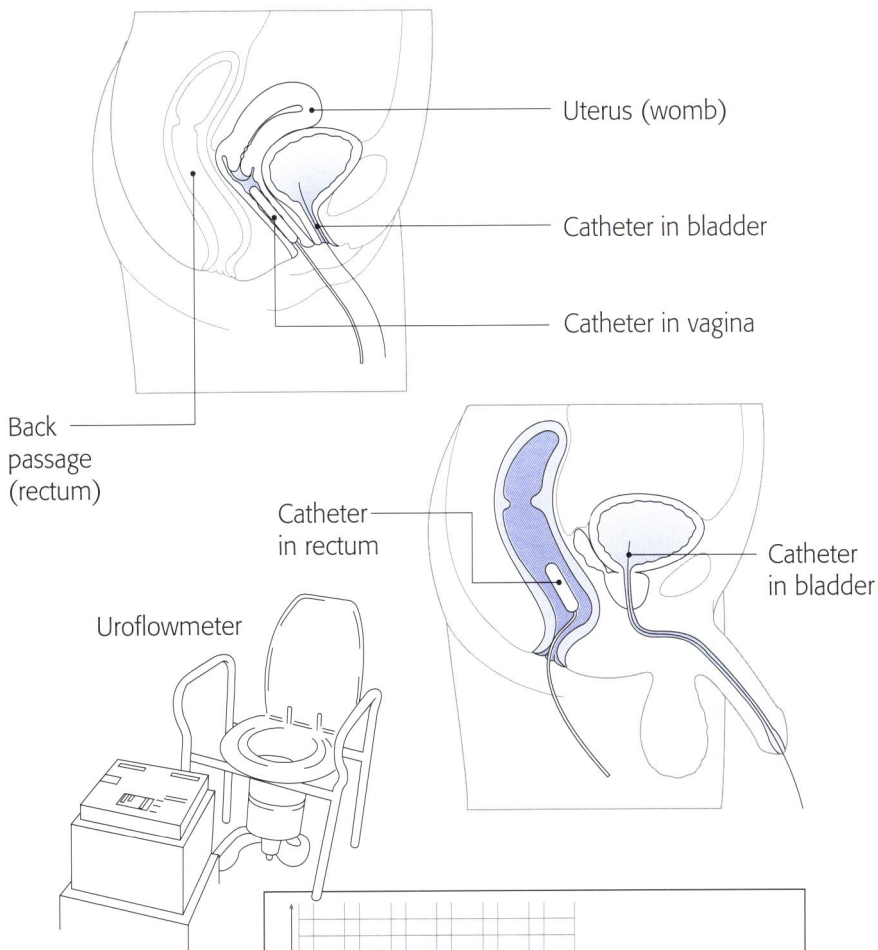

Normal urine flow

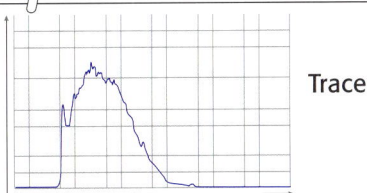

Reduced flow caused by obstruction or by bladder not contracting well

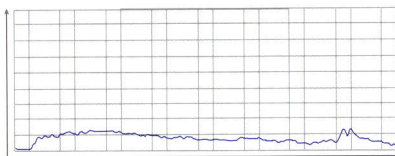

Urethral pressure profilometry

- Incontinence occurs because the pressure in the bladder overcomes the pressure in the urethra – the tube through which the urine is passed.

- Urethral pressure profilometry is a test to measure the pressure inside the bladder and the urethra.

- A catheter is inserted up the urethra and used to fill the bladder with a dilute solution of salt. This catheter is then removed and a special catheter with two sensors is inserted. One of the sensors is used to measure the pressure inside the urethra and the other the pressure inside the bladder. Inserting the special catheter should not be painful as it is quite thin.

- One of the sensors is then slowly withdrawn, so that the pressure along the whole length of the urethra can be measured. It is important that you remain completely still while this is done.

- The procedure is usually repeated to make sure that the readings are accurate. It may also be necessary to repeat the test while you are coughing.

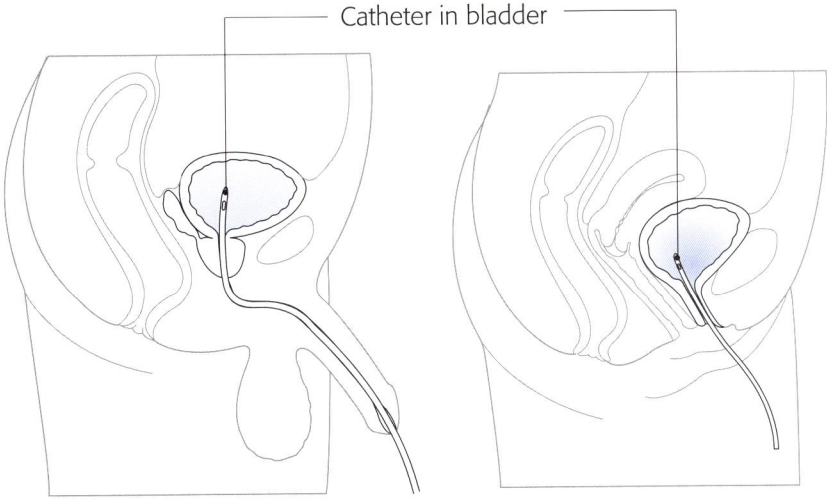

Catheter in bladder

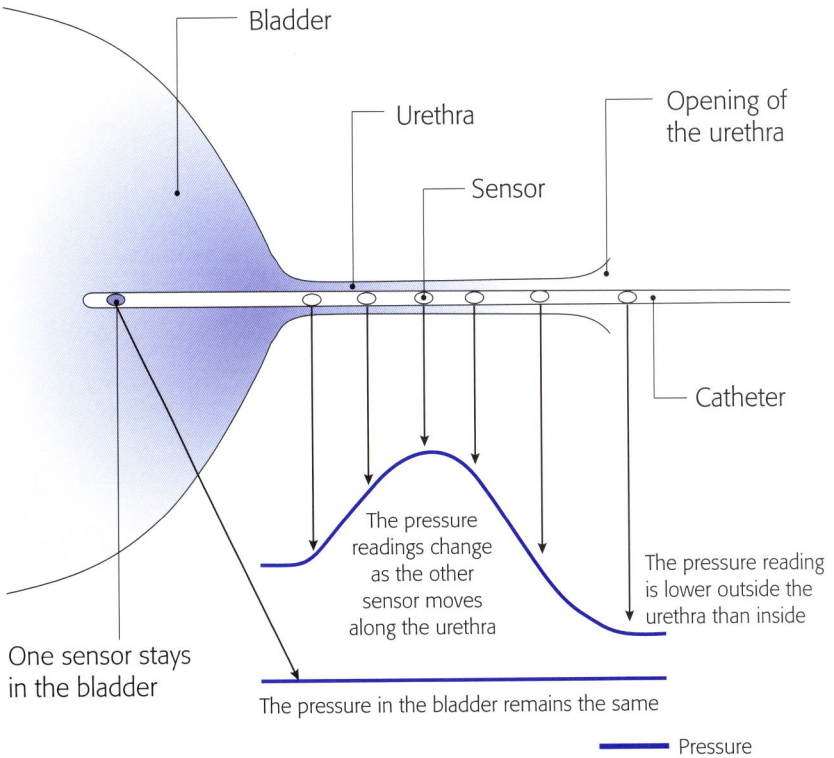

Bladder

Urethra

Opening of the urethra

Sensor

Catheter

The pressure readings change as the other sensor moves along the urethra

The pressure reading is lower outside the urethra than inside

One sensor stays in the bladder

The pressure in the bladder remains the same

Pressure

Urethral sphincter electromyography

- The urethra is surrounded by a ring of muscle. This muscle keeps the urethra closed and prevents urine from leaking out. If the muscle does not work properly, it can lead to incontinence.

- Electromyography or EMG detects the electrical activity in the muscle. This test can be used to find out how well the muscle is working. There are two main types of EMG – surface electrode and needle electrode.

- In surface electrode EMG, the electrode is attached to a catheter. The catheter is then inserted into the urethra. Surface electrode EMG is relatively easy to perform, but it is not as accurate as needle electrode EMG.

- Needle electrode EMG involves inserting a very fine needle through the skin into the muscle around the urethra. This is not as painful as it sounds because the needle is so fine. In women, it can be passed either along the side of the urethra or even through the vagina into the urethra.

- Sometimes, in needle electrode EMG, the patient is asked to pass urine so that the doctor can see how the muscle reacts.

- Both surface and needle electrodes are connected by a wire to an EMG machine. This machine turns the electrical activity picked up by the electrode into a trace that can be seen on the screen or recorded. It is also possible to listen to the activity through a speaker.

Needle electrode EMG

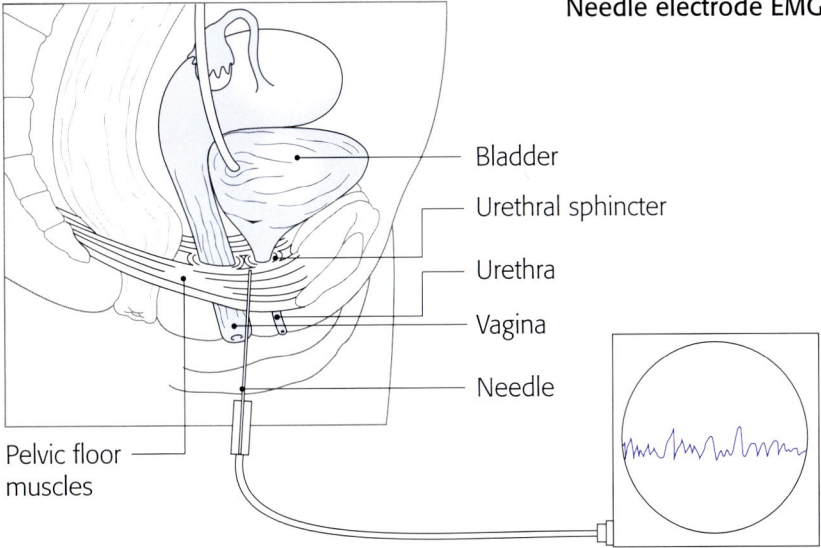

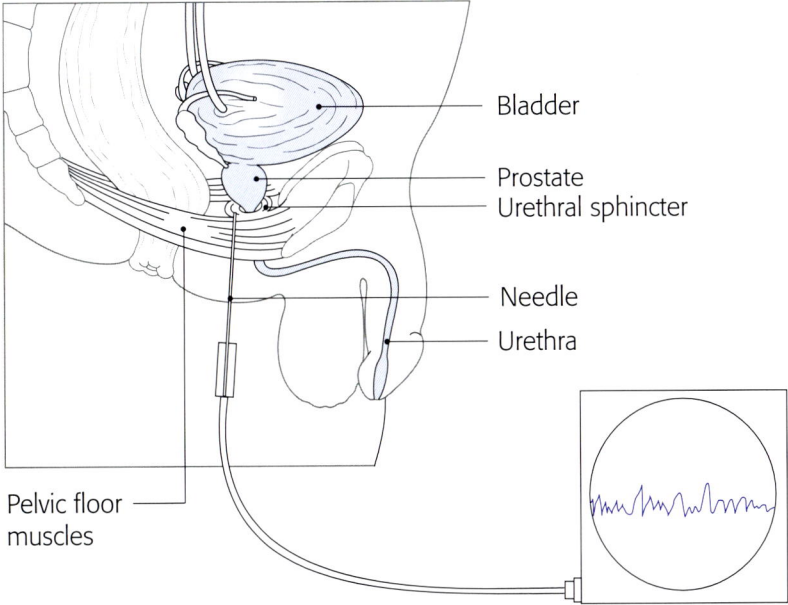

Bladder

Urethral sphincter

Urethra

Vagina

Needle

Pelvic floor muscles

Bladder

Prostate

Urethral sphincter

Needle

Urethra

Pelvic floor muscles

Detrusor instability – symptoms and diagnosis

- In a normal bladder, the bladder muscle contracts only when you decide to urinate, usually when the bladder is full. In detrusor instability or DI, the bladder muscle contracts involuntarily before the bladder is full, and sometimes without warning.

- DI makes you want to go to the toilet more often and more urgently than before. You may also find that you feel a strong desire to pass urine and then suddenly do so without meaning to. This is known as urge incontinence. The symptoms can be triggered by a number of things, such as opening your front door, sex and giggling.

- In many cases, no reason can be found for DI and about 1 in 5 people will be affected in this way at some point in their lives. However, in men, the most common cause of DI is obstruction from the prostate or narrowing of the urethra.

- A series of tests called a urodynamic evaluation will be carried out. You may also be asked to fill in a symptom score sheet or voiding diary for a week. This involves recording every time you go to the toilet, approximately how much urine is passed and how many times you were incontinent and passed urine without meaning to.

- A procedure known as a cystoscopy may also be carried out to check that there are no stones or tumours in the bladder.

Symptom score sheet

FREQUENCY / VOLUME CHART

Name.. Record Number...........................

Date of Start................

Day in Cycle	Sunday		Monday		Tuesday		Wednesday		Thursday		Friday		Saturday	
	IN	OUT	IN	OUT	IN	OUT	IN	OUT	IN	OUT	IN	OUT	IN	OUT
09.00 - 10.00														
10.00 - 11.00														
11.00 - 12.00														
12.00 - 13.00														
13.00 - 14.00														
14.00 - 15.00														
15.00 - 16.00														
16.00 - 17.00														
17.00 - 18.00														
18.00 - 19.00														
19.00 - 20.00														
20.00 - 21.00														
21.00 - 22.00														
22.00 - 23.00														
23.00 - 24.00														
24.00 - 01.00														
01.00 - 02.00														
02.00 - 03.00														
03.00 - 04.00														
04.00 - 05.00														
05.00 - 06.00														
06.00 - 07.00														
07.00 - 08.00														
08.00 - 09.00														
WAKING														
RETIRING														

Enter amount drunk in the "in" column.
Enter volume of urine passed in the "out" column.
Please return this completed chart at your next visit.

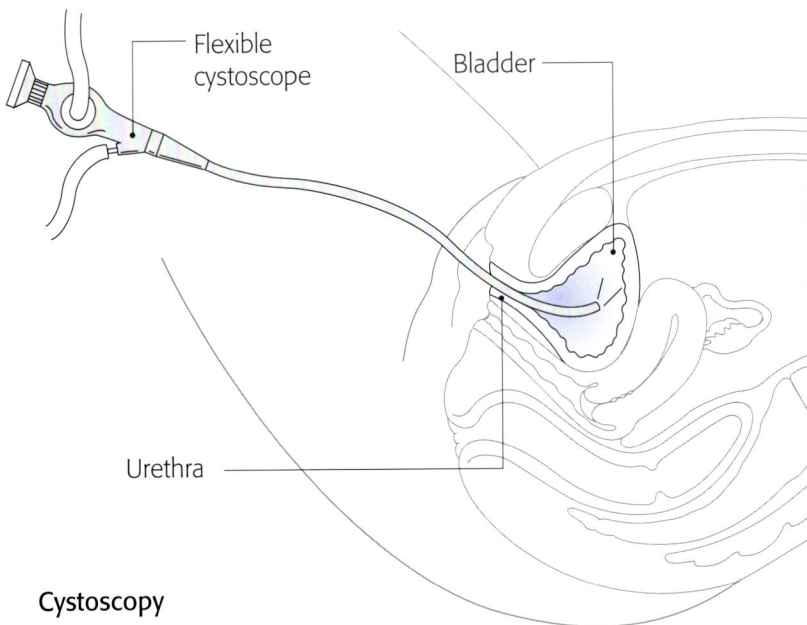

Flexible cystoscope

Bladder

Urethra

Cystoscopy

Detrusor instability – conservative treatment

- Excessive fluid intake is not advisable. If the main problem is night-time trips to the toilet, it may help if you stop drinking in the evening. Avoiding certain types of drink, particularly coffee and alcohol, can also be effective. Some people find that drinking cranberry juice can improve symptoms.

- Bladder training may be useful to increase the volume of fluid that the bladder can hold. This involves trying to 'hold on' for as long as possible when the desire to pass urine occurs. Contracting your pelvic floor muscles can help with this. Gradually, you will find that your bladder can hold larger and larger volumes of urine. The success of this treatment may be shown by noting the number of visits to the toilet and recording the volume of urine passed on each occasion.

- Biofeedback techniques may also be used to help you recognize when unwanted bladder contractions are occurring. A light or buzzer shows when the bladder contracts, and you will be encouraged to try and stop it.

- Some patients find that hypnotherapy or acupuncture can help to improve their symptoms.

- Stretching the bladder may also increase the volume of fluid that the bladder can hold. This involves stretching the bladder by filling it with water under pressure, rather like blowing up a balloon. It is usually done under a general anaesthetic during a procedure called a cystoscopy. Unfortunately, this technique usually provides only short-term relief of symptoms.

Stretching the bladder during cystoscopy

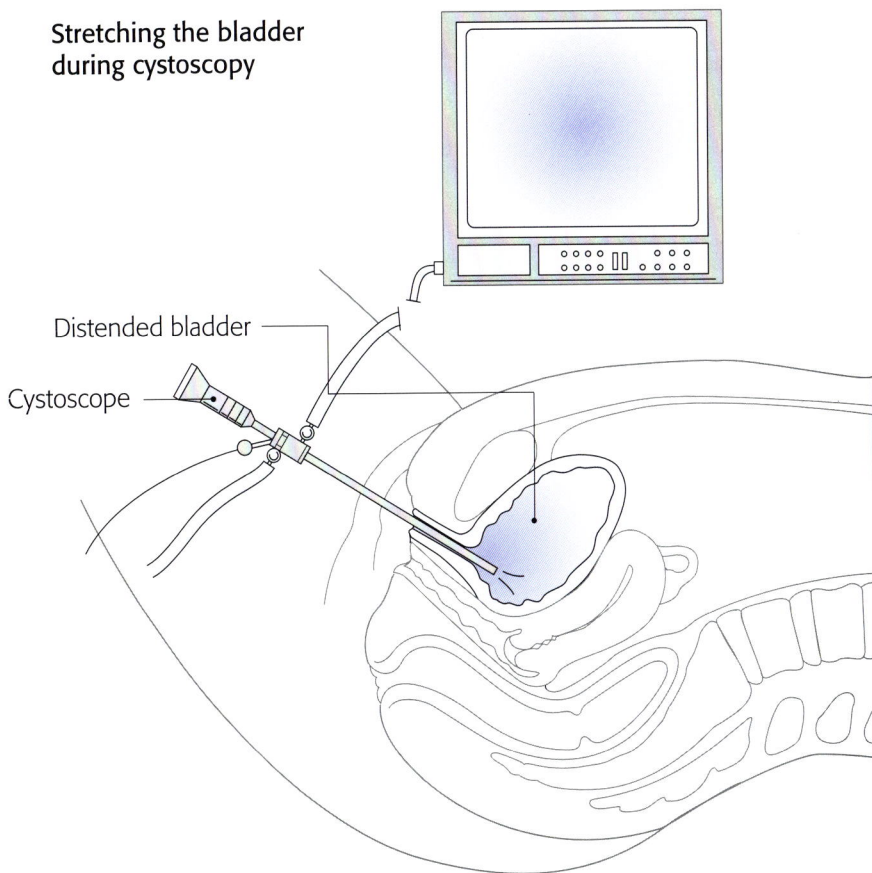

Distended bladder

Cystoscope

Detrusor instability – drug treatment

- Drugs known as diuretics, which are given to remove excess water from the body, can make the symptoms of detrusor instability or DI worse. If this happens, your doctor may prescribe another drug.

- If it is not possible for you to take a different drug, an alternative is to alter the time when the diuretics are taken. Patients bothered by frequent visits to the toilet at night should take their diuretic in the morning and, if necessary, a second dose early in the evening.

- Drugs such as oxybutynin and tolterodine can be used to help stop the unwanted contractions of the bladder. Other drugs that work in this way include flavoxate, nifedipine, imipramine and propantheline. As everyone is different, your doctor may want to try different types and doses of the drugs available.

- The need for frequent visits to the toilet at night, and bedwetting, can be treated with a synthetic hormone called desmopressin. This drug is taken in the form of a nasal spray or a tablet last thing at night.

- Desmopressin must be taken only once a day. Because it effectively stops the kidneys producing urine, when the effect of the drug wears off during the day, more urine is passed out.

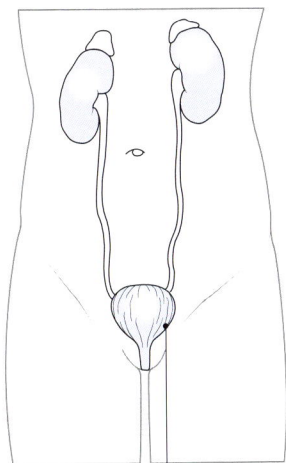

Unwanted contractions
of the bladder

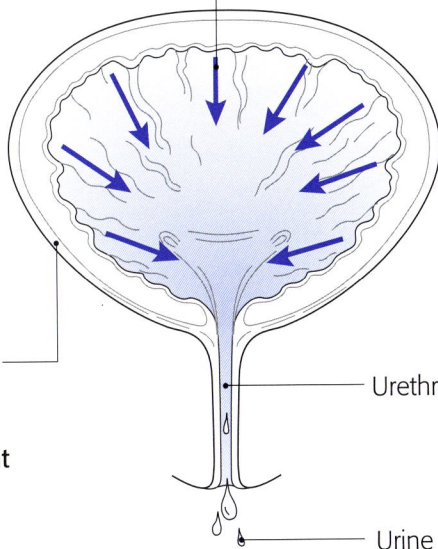

Bladder

Urethra

Before treatment

Urine

After treatment

Bladder contracts
less often and can
hold more urine

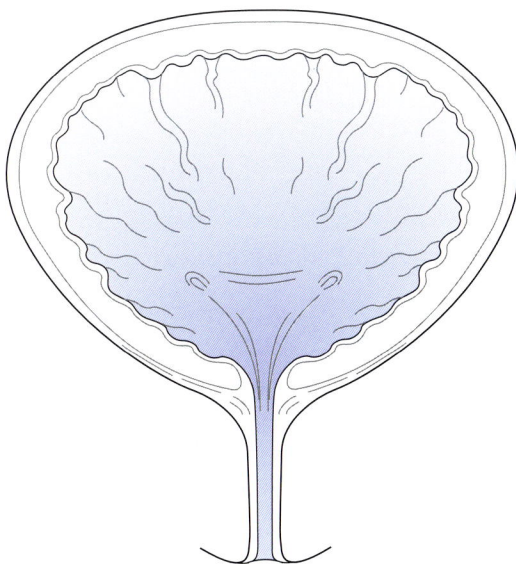

Detrusor instability – containment and devices

- Waterproof underwear that holds absorbent pads is available. This option is suitable for patients with mild-to-moderate incontinence. Your continence advisor or specialist nurse can help you choose the best product for you.

- Another alternative for men is an external device, such as the penile sheath or penile clamp. The penile sheath can be attached via a tube to a bag, which fits neatly around the leg. These external devices do not have to be used permanently and many patients use them only when they cannot reach a toilet quickly, or at night-time.

- For some patients, a permanent urethral catheter is the best solution. Although this will usually control the incontinence, it may cause discomfort, repeated urinary tract infections and/or become encrusted with salts found in the urine. Replacing the catheter every 3 months can help to avoid some of these problems.

- Some patients prefer to attach the catheter to a valve device, rather than a catheter bag. The valve stops the urine flowing out. However, bag drainage is usually preferable at night.

- A permanent suprapubic catheter is more comfortable than a urethral catheter, especially for men. It can be inserted under a local or general anaesthetic and will need to be changed about every 3 months. Patients do not usually need an anaesthetic when the catheter is changed. For this catheter to work successfully, some patients will require another operation to close the bladder neck.

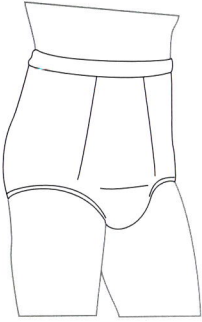

Waterproof
underwear

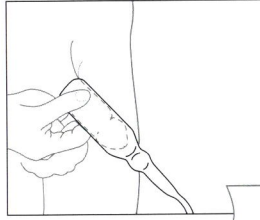

Penile sheath

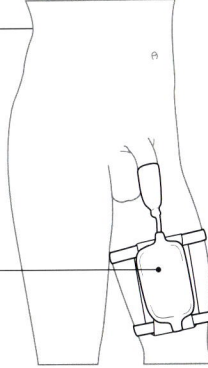

Leg bag

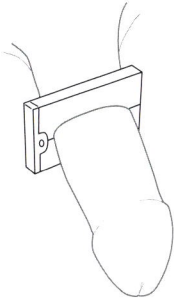

Penile clamp

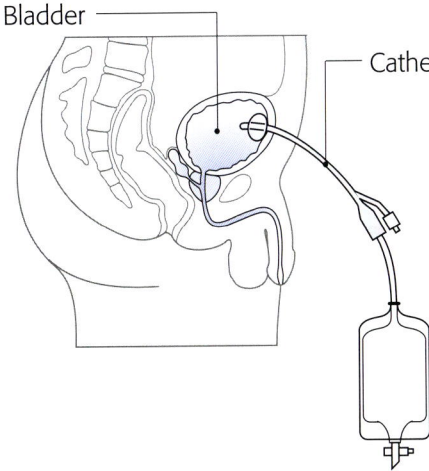

Bladder

Catheter

Suprapubic catheter

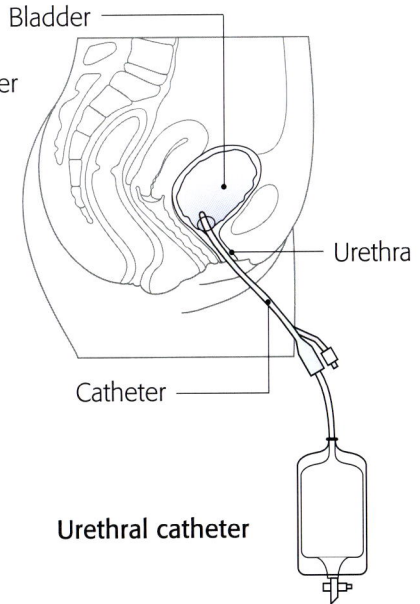

Bladder

Urethra

Catheter

Urethral catheter

Detrusor instability – surgical treatments

- Detrusor myectomy and clam or Bramble cystoplasty are two types of operation that can be carried out to treat detrusor instability or DI that has not responded to other simpler treatments.

- Detrusor myectomy involves making a cut in the lower abdomen and removing much of the bladder muscle.

- The operation is carried out under a general anaesthetic and takes about 2 hours. You will need to stay in hospital for several days.

- The clam or Bramble cystoplasty involves opening the bladder like a clam and inserting a piece of intestine to enlarge the bladder. This weakens the bladder contractions and increases the volume of urine that the bladder can hold.

- Clam or Bramble cystoplasty is carried out under a general anaesthetic and takes about 2 hours. The average hospital stay is variable, but complete recovery may take 3–4 months.

- During both types of operation, a catheter is passed up the urethra to drain off the urine while the bladder heals. This will be removed after about 1 week.

- After the operation, the bladder will not contract to push the urine out as well as it does normally, and you may need to learn to pass a catheter up the urethra on a regular basis to empty the bladder fully.

Incision

Urethra

Bladder

Outer muscle layer

Urethra

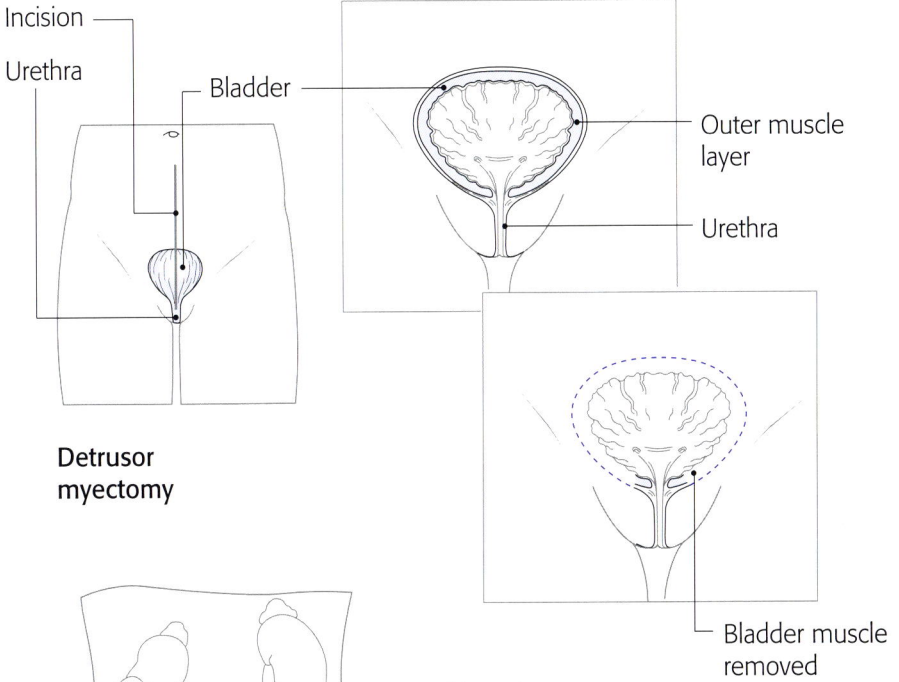

Detrusor myectomy

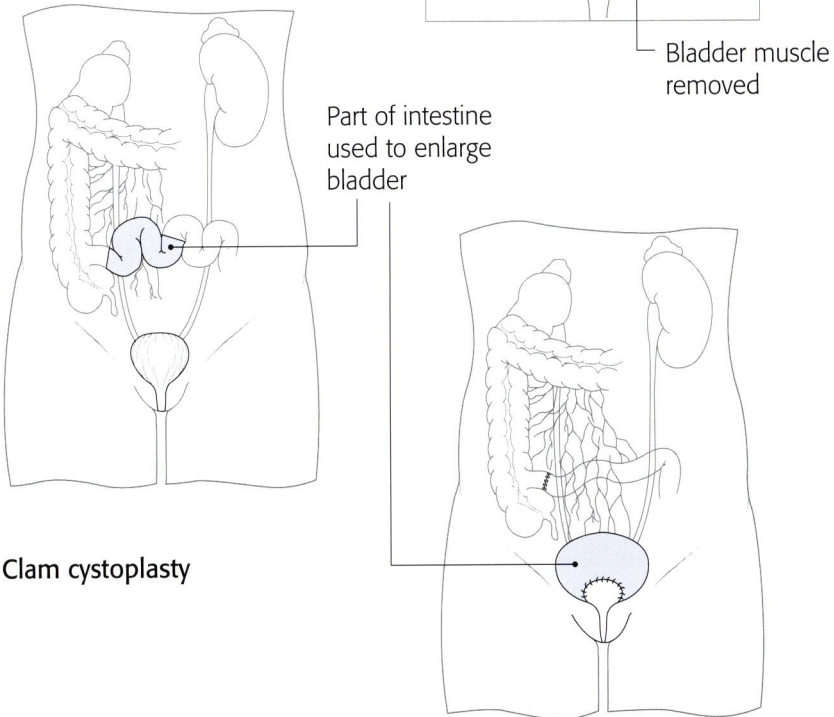

Bladder muscle removed

Part of intestine used to enlarge bladder

Clam cystoplasty

Detrusor instability – urinary diversion

- When other surgical or drug treatments for incontinence caused by detrusor instability have been unsuccessful, an operation called a urinary diversion may be considered.

- The procedure involves making an artificial opening called a stoma in the abdominal wall to drain the urine from the bladder. The two main ways of doing this are called the ileal conduit and continent diversion. Both operations are carried out under a general anaesthetic.

- The ileal conduit involves using a piece of intestine to connect the ureters to the stoma. A bag can then be attached to the stoma to collect the urine.

- The operation usually takes about 2 hours. During the operation, small tubes are placed in each of the ureters to hold them open. These are usually removed 1 week later. The length of your hospital stay will depend on your post-operative progress. When you are well enough, you will be taught how to care for your stoma and change the bags.

- A continent diversion avoids the need for a bag. A small pouch is formed from a piece of intestine to act as a reservoir for the urine in place of the bladder. Another piece of intestine is then used to connect the pouch to an opening in the abdominal wall. Special valves may be put in the pouch to prevent urine from going back up the ureters and into the kidneys, or leaking from the opening.

- The operation takes 2–3 hours. When you are well enough, you will be taught how to drain the urine from the pouch. This will need to be done 4–5 times a day.

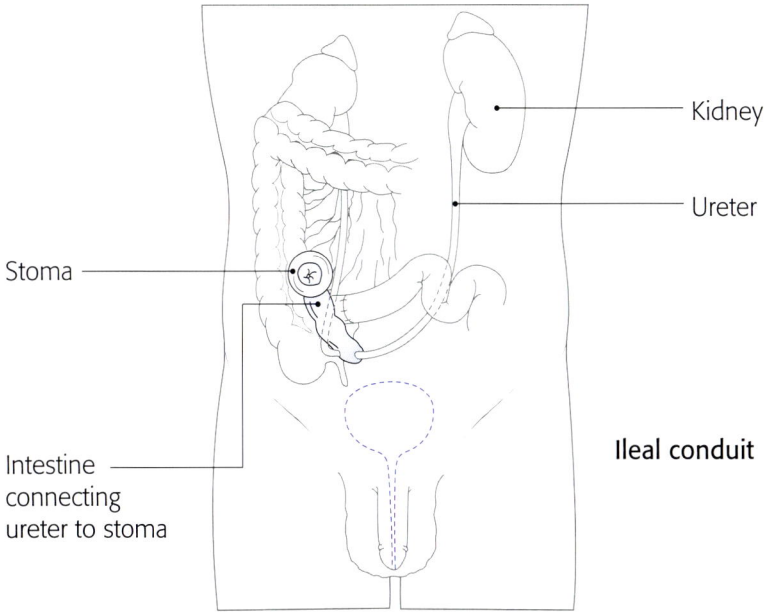

Kidney

Ureter

Stoma

Ileal conduit

Intestine
connecting
ureter to stoma

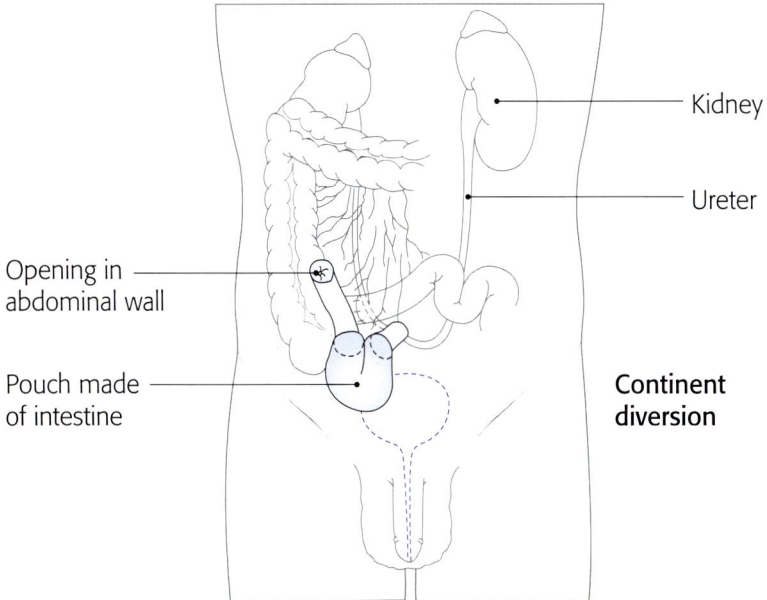

Kidney

Ureter

Opening in
abdominal wall

Pouch made
of intestine

Continent
diversion

Stress incontinence

- Stress incontinence describes leakage of urine when you cough, sneeze, strain or as a consequence of a similar activity. It is particularly common in women. Genuine stress incontinence (diagnosed by urodynamic investigations) occurs when the bladder neck and the other mechanisms that act to hold urine in the bladder are not working properly.

- The neck of the bladder is much stronger in men than in women, though it can become weakened following surgery on the prostate. It is less important for continence in women, and it does tend to weaken with age.

- Another mechanism, the urethral sphincter, is very important for continence in women, less so in men. It comprises the muscle that surrounds the urethra and its attachments to the pelvic floor muscles. For the urethral sphincter mechanism to work properly, the tissue that supports the pelvic floor, known as the fascia, has to be intact.

- After childbirth, the fascia may become disrupted so that the bladder neck starts to lose its support. Over time, the defect becomes more pronounced so that the unsupported bladder neck moves excessively downwards during activity, resulting in urine leakage. This movement of the bladder neck is called hypermobility.

- The intrinsic urethral sphincter mechanism may also fail. In men, this can occur after prostate surgery; in women, it can occur after surgery for incontinence, with age or after childbirth.

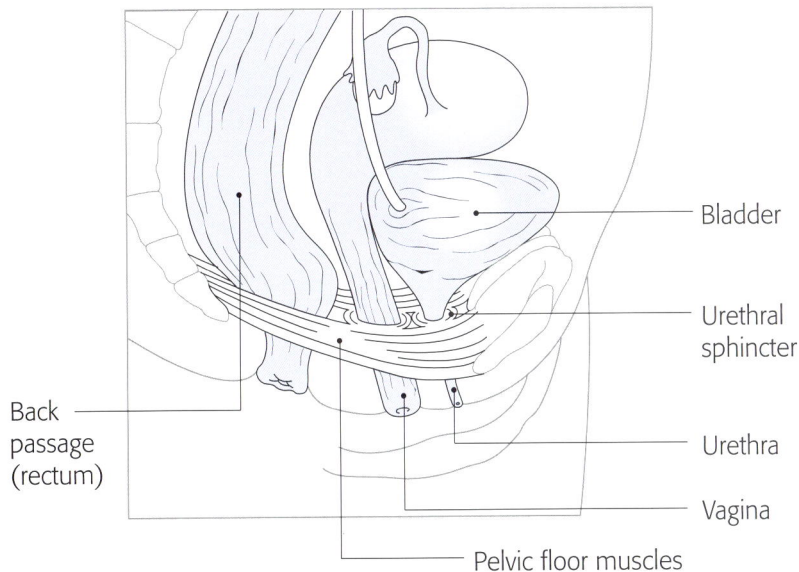

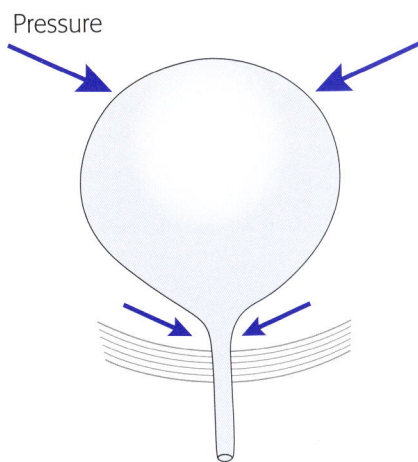

Bladder

Urethral sphincter

Urethra

Back passage (rectum)

Vagina

Pelvic floor muscles

Pressure

Pressure

Urine

Continence
Activities cause increased pressure in the abdomen. The pressure is transmitted to the urethra and the bladder.

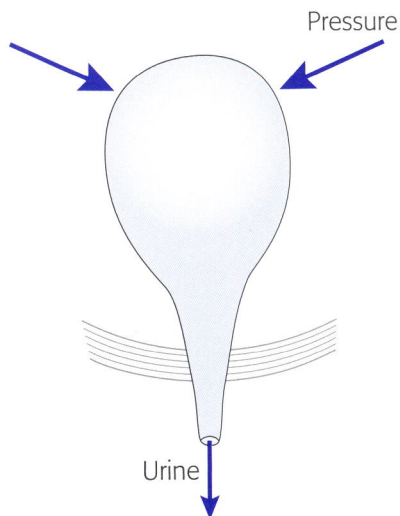

Incontinence
Activities cause increased pressure in the abdomen. The bladder neck moves down so all the pressure is transmitted to the bladder

Treatment of genuine stress incontinence

- The most common treatments for genuine stress incontinence involve surgery or techniques to 'train' the pelvic floor muscles. The aim of both approaches is to stabilize the bladder neck.

- Surgery may be performed through the vagina and/or through an incision in the abdomen. Your surgery will permanently change the anatomy of your bladder neck support in an attempt to make the bladder neck more stable. Your doctor will discuss exactly what is involved with you.

- Other treatments involve strengthening the pelvic floor muscles that support the bladder neck, and increasing the speed with which they can contract. For example, you might be given a set of exercises to train your pelvic floor muscles.

- Pelvic floor exercises, sometimes called Kegels, involve contracting or 'pulling up' the muscles of your pelvic floor. Your exercise plan may require you to contract your muscles for as long as possible or to carry out a series of short contractions. Pelvic floor exercises need to be practised every day.

- It is sometimes difficult to identify your pelvic floor muscles. Your doctor may be able to offer you a technique called biofeedback, which allows you to see on a TV screen that you are contracting the right muscles, and allows you to monitor the strength of the contractions. Alternatively, your doctor may examine you vaginally while you perform the exercises to check that you are doing them correctly.

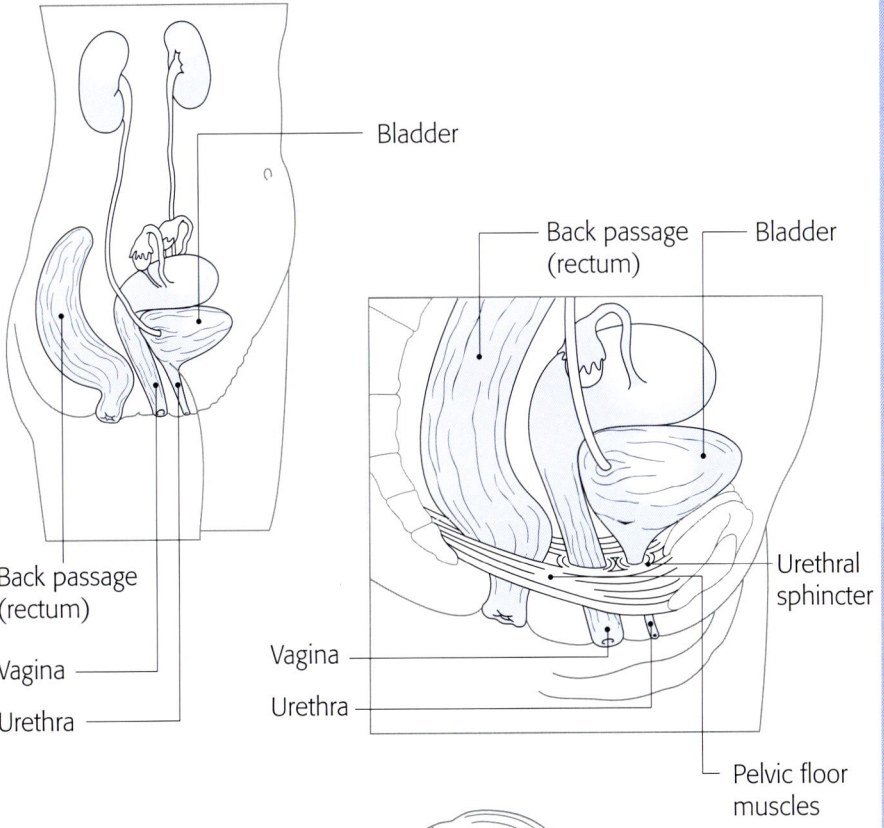

Bladder

Back passage
(rectum)

Bladder

Back passage
(rectum)

Vagina

Urethra

Urethral
sphincter

Vagina

Urethra

Pelvic floor
muscles

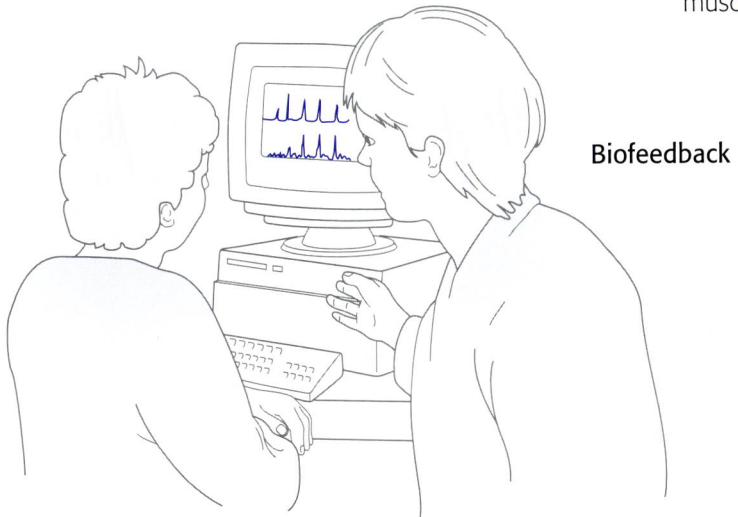

Biofeedback

Vaginal cones

- Vaginal cones are designed to help you contract your pelvic floor muscles without contracting your abdominal muscles.

- Some vaginal cones come in a set of five of the same size but with different weights. Others come as two outer casings that can be unscrewed and filled with different weights. Both types have a thread attached, so they can be easily removed like a tampon. You should start with the lightest cone and work up towards the heaviest cone.

- The cone is inserted into the top of the vagina leaving the thread outside. When you stand up, you will need to contract your pelvic floor muscles to keep the cone inside the vagina. If you strain and increase the pressure inside your abdomen, like you do when passing a stool, the cone will be pushed out.

- You should walk around for about 15 minutes with this weight of cone. When you can manage this easily, you should repeat the process with the next size up. The more you use cones, the better you will get, but you should practise every day.

- This process is basically weight-training of the pelvic floor and, though simple, it is quite effective.

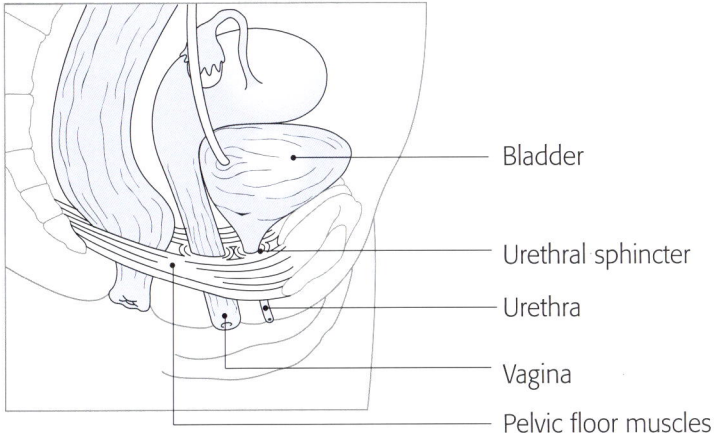

— Bladder

— Urethral sphincter

— Urethra

— Vagina

— Pelvic floor muscles

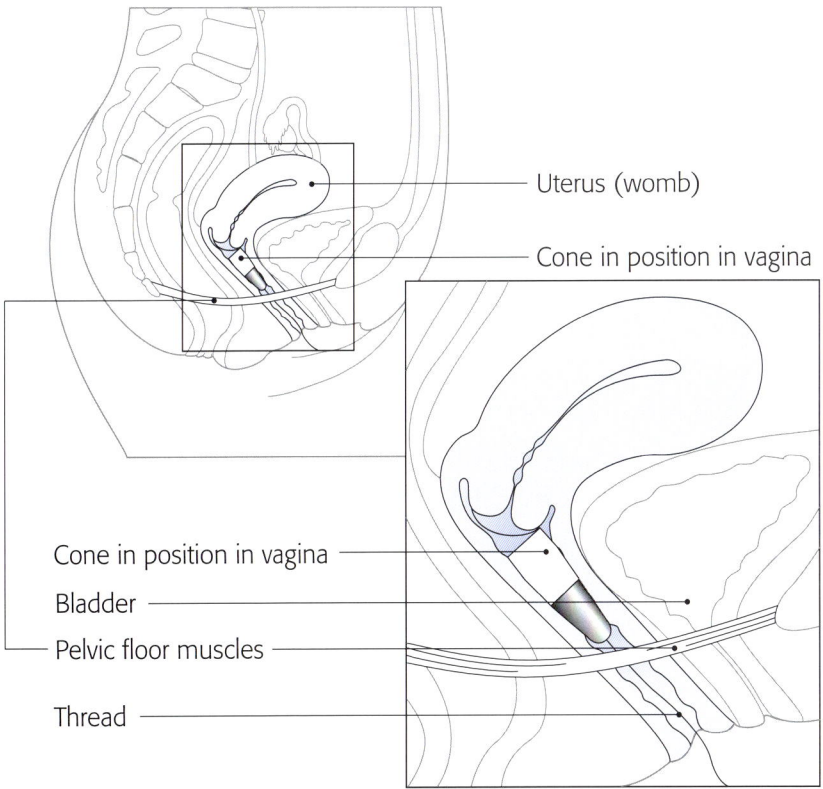

— Uterus (womb)

— Cone in position in vagina

Cone in position in vagina —

Bladder —

— Pelvic floor muscles

Thread —

Colposuspension

- Colposuspension is an effective operation for curing genuine stress incontinence, which is caused by a weakness of bladder neck support.

- The operation involves stabilizing the bladder neck by inserting several stitches through the tissue on each side, and attaching them to a ligament on the pelvic bone.

- The operation is performed under a general or spinal anaesthetic and takes 1/2–2 hours.

- This is a major operation that requires a bikini-line incision.

- The average hospital stay is 2–7 days and normal activities can usually be resumed within 6–8 weeks.

- After the operation, you may need to have a catheter for about a week, sometimes longer.

- Occasionally, the surgeon may be able to carry out this operation using 'key-hole' surgery. This has the advantage of requiring a few smaller incisions, causing less discomfort and enabling a faster recovery. Some surgeons still consider this to be experimental.

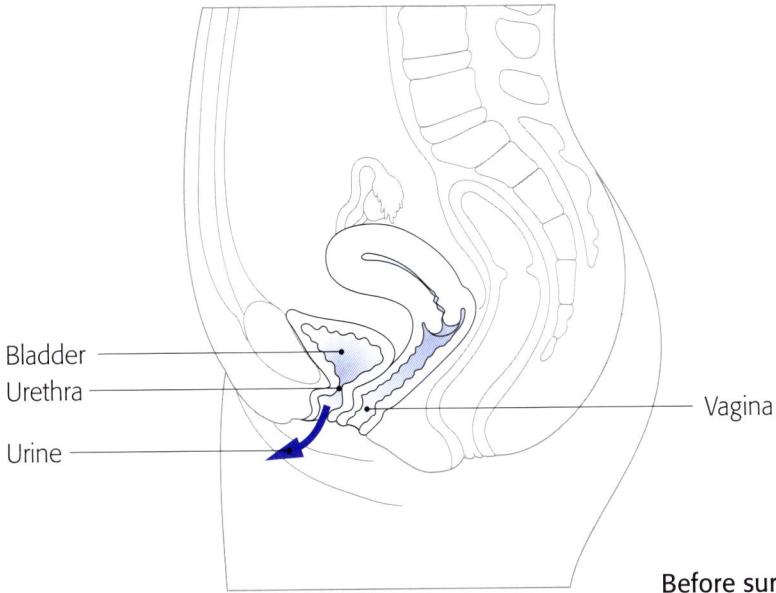

Bladder

Urethra

Urine

Vagina

Before surgery

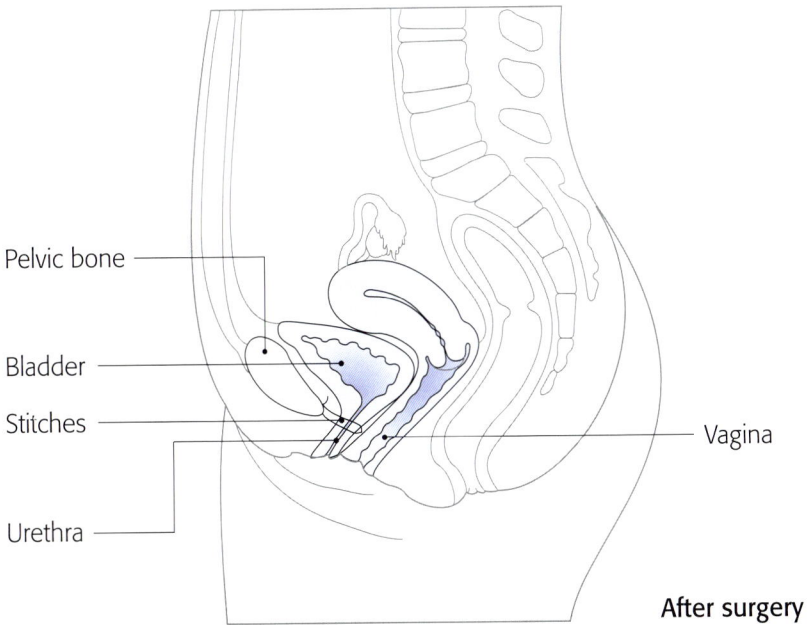

Pelvic bone

Bladder

Stitches

Urethra

Vagina

After surgery

Anterior (cystocele) repair

- This operation is carried out for prolapse and/or incontinence.

- The bladder and/or urethra can 'drop' or prolapse into the front wall of the vagina and this can lead to incontinence.

- Repair of the prolapse involves removing a piece of vaginal skin, then stitching the bladder and urethra back into their normal positions and repairing the vagina.

- The operation is performed through the vagina and no scars will be visible afterwards. It is performed under a general or spinal anaesthetic and takes 40–60 minutes.

- During the operation, a catheter may be passed up the urethra into the bladder to drain off the urine. A pack of gauze may also be inserted into the vagina to prevent bleeding after the operation. The gauze will be removed the next day.

- There will be some discomfort following surgery, but less than with abdominal operations. This will be controlled with painkillers.

- The hospital stay is 1–6 days, but you will need to rest at home afterwards. Normal activities can usually be resumed within 6 weeks.

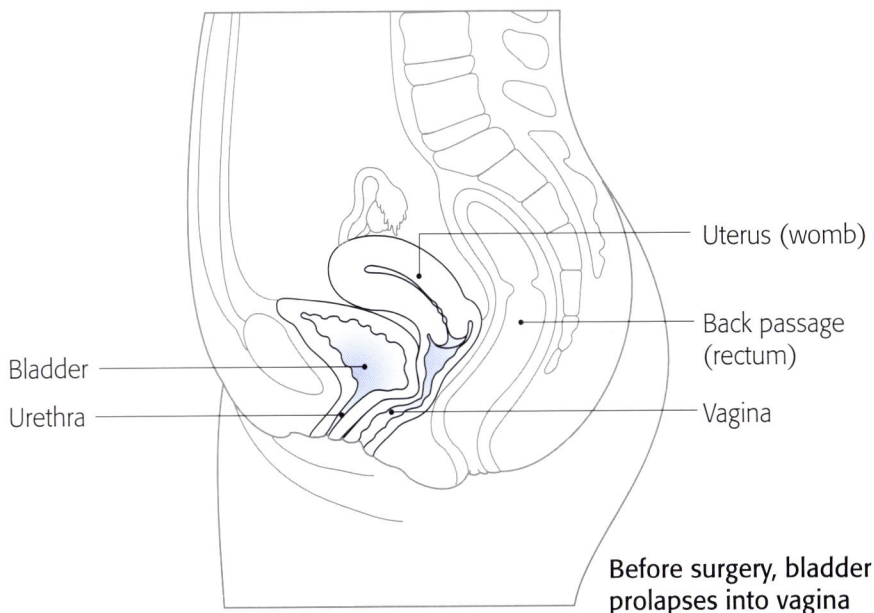

Uterus (womb)

Back passage
(rectum)

Bladder

Urethra

Vagina

**Before surgery, bladder
prolapses into vagina**

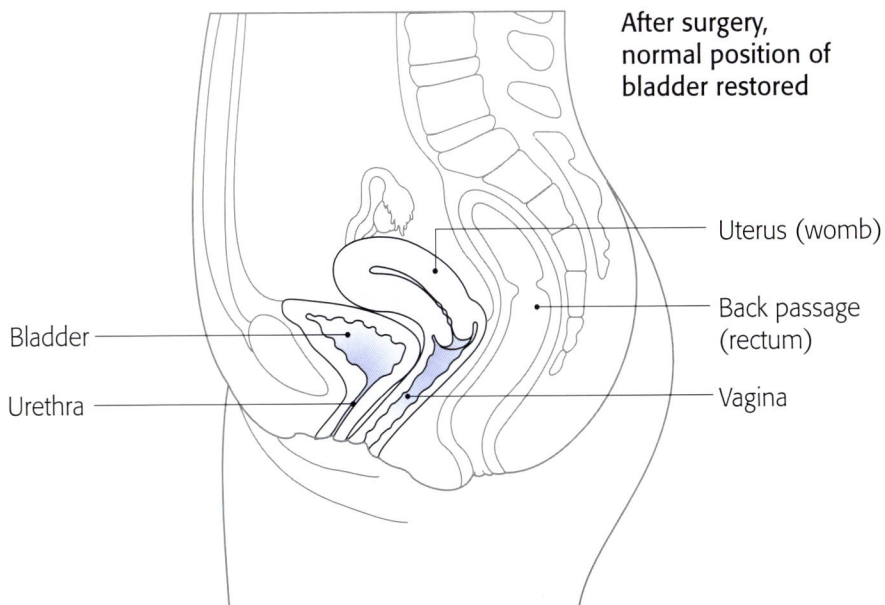

**After surgery,
normal position of
bladder restored**

Uterus (womb)

Back passage
(rectum)

Bladder

Urethra

Vagina

Needle suspension procedures

- Needle suspension procedures are used to treat incontinence that is caused by a weakness of bladder neck support. The operations are often called by the name of the surgeon who invented them, for example, Peyrera, Stamey, Gittes, Raz and Musnai.

- The operation is performed under a general or spinal anaesthetic and takes under 1 hour.

- Two small incisions are made in the abdomen and another is made in the vagina. A stitch is placed on either side of the neck of the bladder and pulled through to just above the pubic bone. The stitches are then pulled up to support the neck of the bladder. They can be tied over the lining and muscle of the abdominal wall or attached to a bone anchor screw.

- The average hospital stay is 1–3 days and normal activities can usually be resumed within 6 weeks, but heavy lifting should always be avoided.

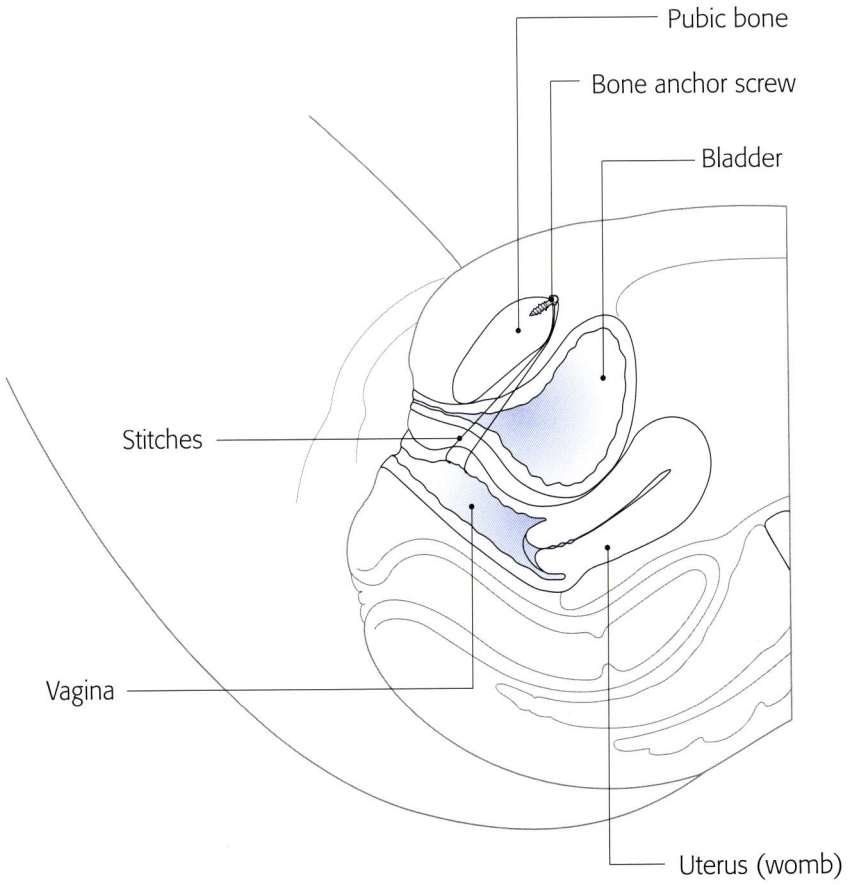

Pubic bone

Bone anchor screw

Bladder

Stitches

Vagina

Uterus (womb)

Sling procedures

- A sling procedure is an operation used to treat incontinence caused by weakness of bladder neck support, or by failure of the intrinsic urethral sphincter mechanism. A sling procedure is often carried out if other treatments have not been successful.

- A small incision is made in the vagina and a strip of material is threaded through underneath the urethra. The material is then picked through another small incision in the abdomen and tied to a ligament inside the pelvis or to the lining of the abdominal wall.

- In patients with incontinence due to a weakness of bladder neck support, the aim is to support the bladder neck with the sling. If the incontinence is due to a weak urethral sphincter, the aim is to stop leakage by compressing the urethra.

- The operation can be performed under a local or general anaesthetic and takes 1–2 hours.

- Difficulties with passing urine are quite common after this operation and you are likely to need a catheter for 1–3 weeks.

- The average hospital stay is 1–7 days and normal activities can usually be resumed within 6 weeks.

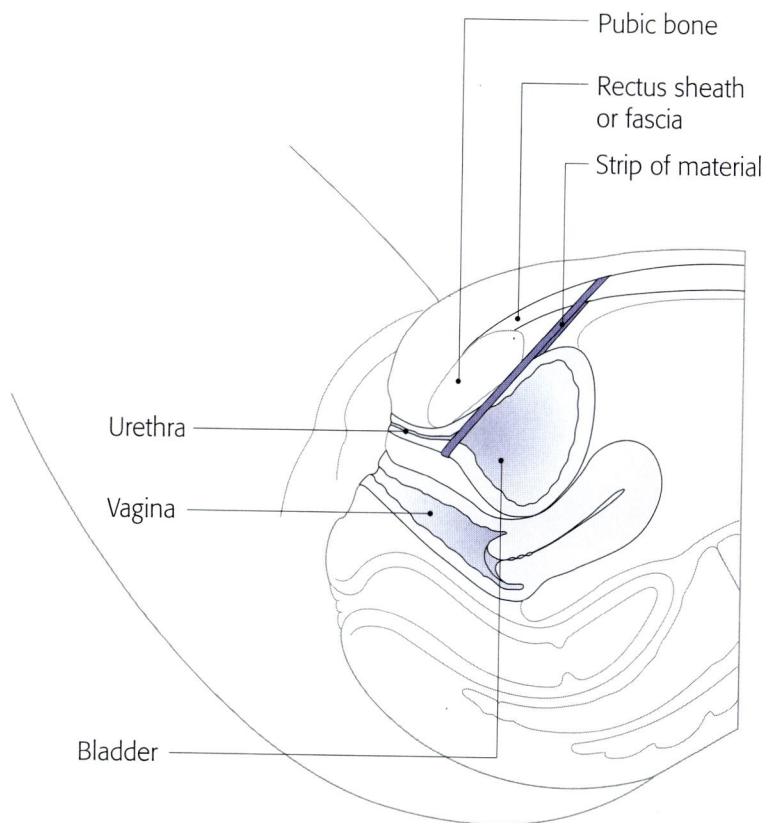

Pubic bone

Rectus sheath or fascia

Strip of material

Urethra

Vagina

Bladder

Injectable agents

- Injectable agents are used to treat incontinence caused by failure of the intrinsic urethral sphincter mechanism.

- Failure of the intrinsic urethral sphincter mechanism results in the bladder neck remaining open. However, substances can be injected into the neck of the bladder to close it again.

- The substances used are not harmful. One of the most commonly used substances is called collagen, and is very similar to the collagen used in cosmetic surgery. Other substances that may be used include the patient's own fat tissue, usually from the abdomen, and special types of plastic.

- The operation is performed under a local, spinal or general anaesthetic and takes about 20 minutes. It can be performed as a day-case procedure.

- A thin 'telescope' called a cystoscope is passed up the urethra. In all men and some women, the substance is injected into the bladder neck using a fine needle introduced through the cystoscope. An alternative in women is to pass the needle up beside the urethra and inject the substance into the bladder neck until it can be seen to close through the cystoscope.

- The injection may need to be repeated if the best effect was not achieved with the first injection or the effect of the injection wears off after a period of time. Many people have more than one injection.

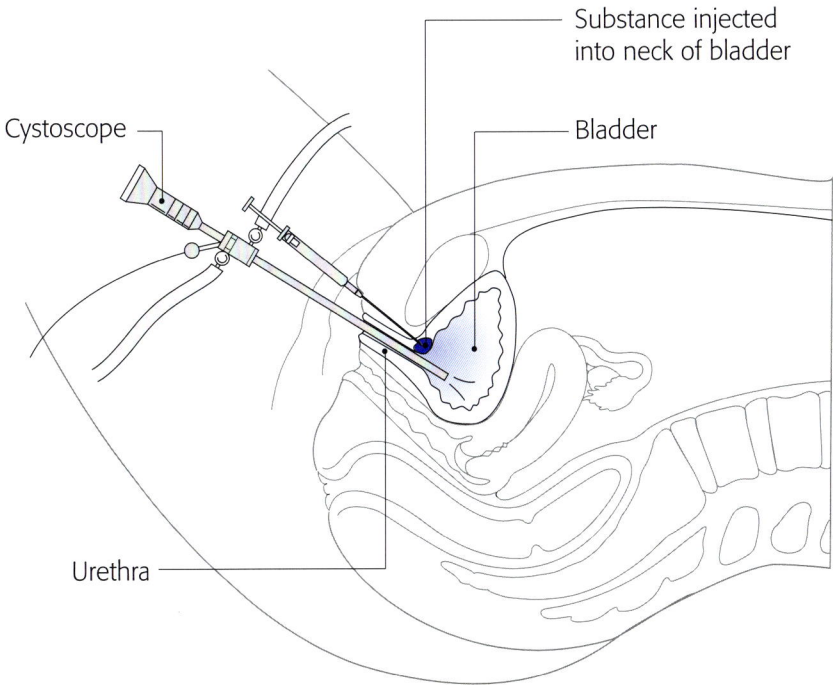

21

Substance injected into neck of bladder

Cystoscope

Bladder

Urethra

Pessaries and devices

- Several devices are available to help control incontinence. These can be useful for patients who are not fit or ready for surgery, or who do not wish to have surgery. They can also be useful for patients who experience problems only in certain situations, such as when doing strenuous exercise.

- These devices can be divided into three groups – those that are placed in the vagina, those that are attached outside the urethra, and those that are put inside the urethra.

- Devices that are placed in the vagina work by pressing on the urethra. This closes the urethra and prevents urine from leaking. The simplest vaginal device looks like a large tampon, which is easy to insert and remove. Some devices can be left in place even while passing urine or having sex. Others need to be adjusted just before urinating and then readjusted again afterwards.

- The amount of incontinence can also be controlled by using a little cap or adhesive patch that is fixed to the opening of the urethra. As these devices are not placed inside the urethra, they do not appear to cause any harm, but some patients may experience a little local irritation.

- Devices that are inserted into the urethra tend to be more difficult to use and can lead to urinary tract infections. They need to be removed for urination. This means that several devices are used each day, which can be expensive. These devices may, however, be the best solution for some patients.

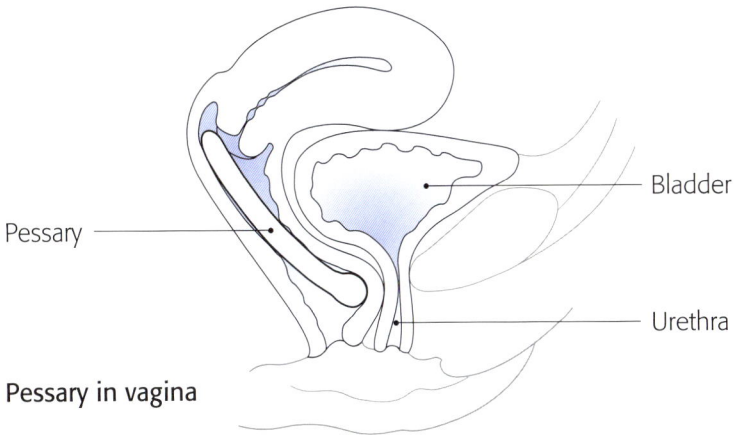

22

Pessary

Bladder

Urethra

Pessary in vagina

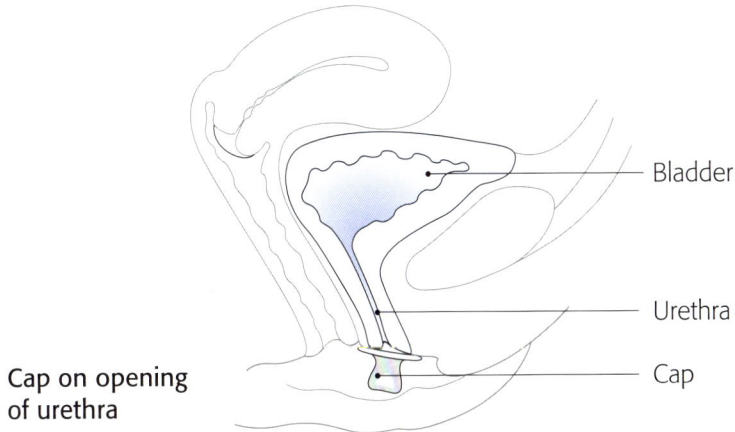

Bladder

Urethra

Cap

Cap on opening of urethra

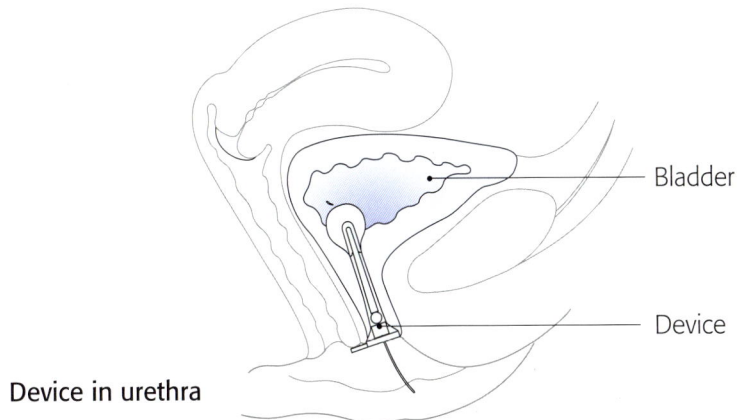

Bladder

Device

Device in urethra

Hormonal therapy

- Stress incontinence is very common at the time of the menopause.

- Oestrogen therapy is often used as part of the treatment for stress incontinence, and is also often given before surgery to strengthen the tissues.

- Oestrogen therapy can be given as tablets, as a skin patch or as a hormone implant. It may also be given as a vaginal ring, or as a cream or tablet that is inserted into the vagina.

- Oestrogen treatment alone is not always effective and another drug called an alpha-agonist may be given at the same time.

- Phenoxybenzamine is an example of an alpha-agonist. It 'tones up' the muscle of the urethra, especially when it is given with oestrogen.

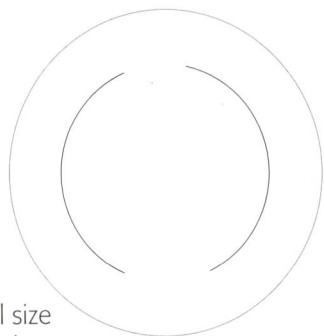

23

Actual size
of patch

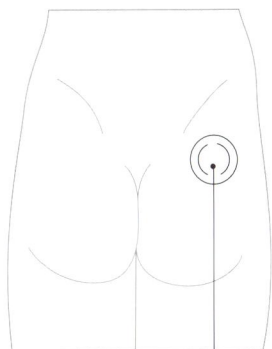

Patch in position

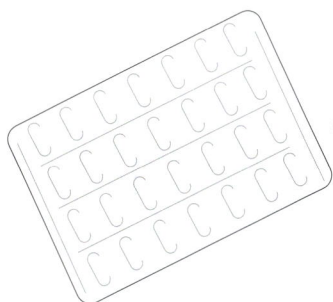

Oestrogen tablets

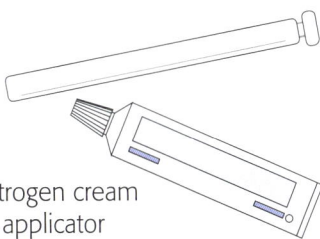

Oestrogen cream
and applicator

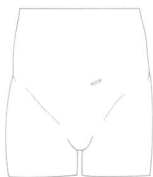

Common position for hormone implants

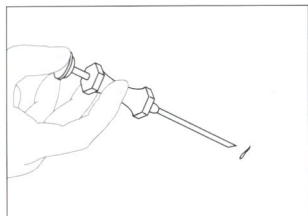

An introducer is used
to insert the implant

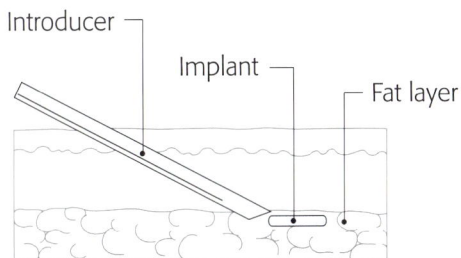

Introducer

Implant

Fat layer

The implant lies in the
fat layer under the skin

Genital prolapse

- A prolapse is when an organ 'drops out' of its normal position. There are several different types of genital prolapse, which can involve the uterus (womb), the bladder, the back passage (rectum) or the bowel. They are all due to pelvic floor weakness.

- Prolapses can be treated by surgery or with pessaries. Prolapse operations are usually performed through the vagina, though sometimes they are performed through an incision in the abdomen.

- In most prolapse operations, the organs are stitched back into their normal position. If the uterus is involved, it can be removed in a hysterectomy procedure. An alternative for women who wish to remain fertile is to put the uterus back into position by shortening the cervix. This procedure is called the Manchester operation.

- A pessary is a device that is inserted into the vagina to hold the organs in their correct positions.

- The choice of pessary will depend on the type of prolapse. Most pessaries are made of 'tissue-friendly' silicone.

- Pessaries come in different sizes and selecting the correct size is important. Your pessary may need to be changed for one of a different size if you gain or lose weight.

- Postmenopausal women will also be given vaginal oestrogen as a cream. Without vaginal oestrogen, the pessary is more likely to cause ulcers on the vagina, which can cause discharge, and even bleeding and infection.

24

Before surgery

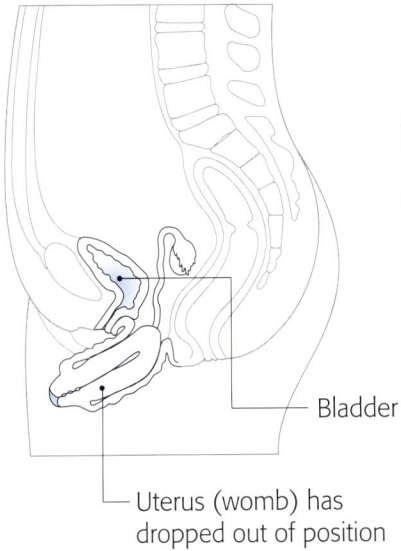

After surgery

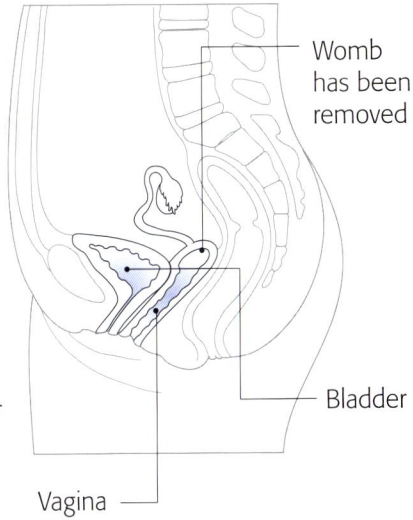

Womb
has been
removed

Bladder

Bladder

Uterus (womb) has
dropped out of position

Vagina

Without pessary

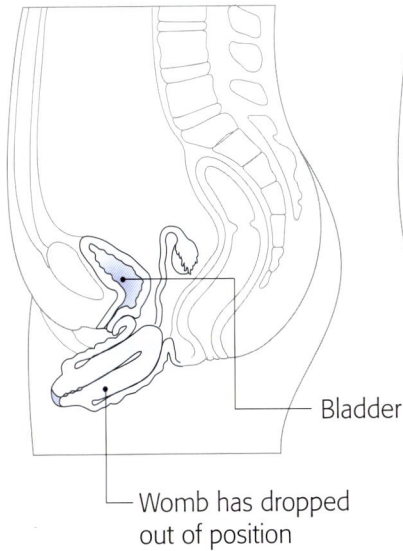

With pessary

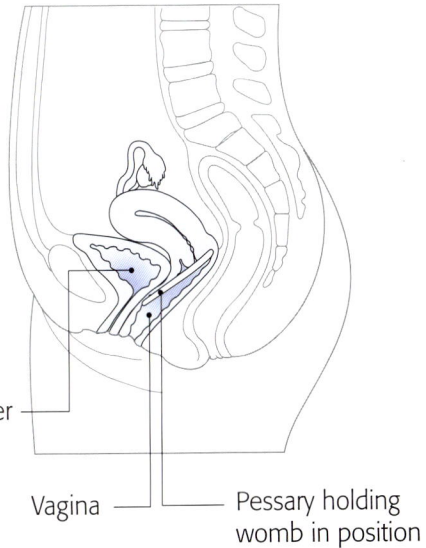

Bladder

Womb has dropped
out of position

Vagina

Pessary holding
womb in position

Bladder cancer

- There are several different types of bladder cancer. The most common tumour is called transitional cell carcinoma. Other less common tumours are squamous cell carcinoma, adenocarcinoma and sarcoma.

- Factors that may increase the likelihood of bladder cancer developing include smoking, exposure to chemicals and infection with some tropical parasites.

- The treatment of bladder cancer depends on the type of tumour and how far it has spread.

- Early disease is usually removed in a procedure called a cystoscopy. This enables the bladder lining to be examined and any areas affected by the tumour to be removed.

- For more advanced superficial disease, a catheter is used to fill the bladder with a special solution containing anti-cancer drugs. The drugs are left in the bladder for about half an hour.

- Tumours that have invaded the bladder wall are best treated with an operation called a cystectomy. This involves removing the bladder. The bladder can be reconstructed or the urine diverted through an opening in the abdominal wall.

- Occasionally, in elderly or unfit patients, advanced bladder cancer is treated with radiotherapy. However, an operation on the bladder may be necessary later.

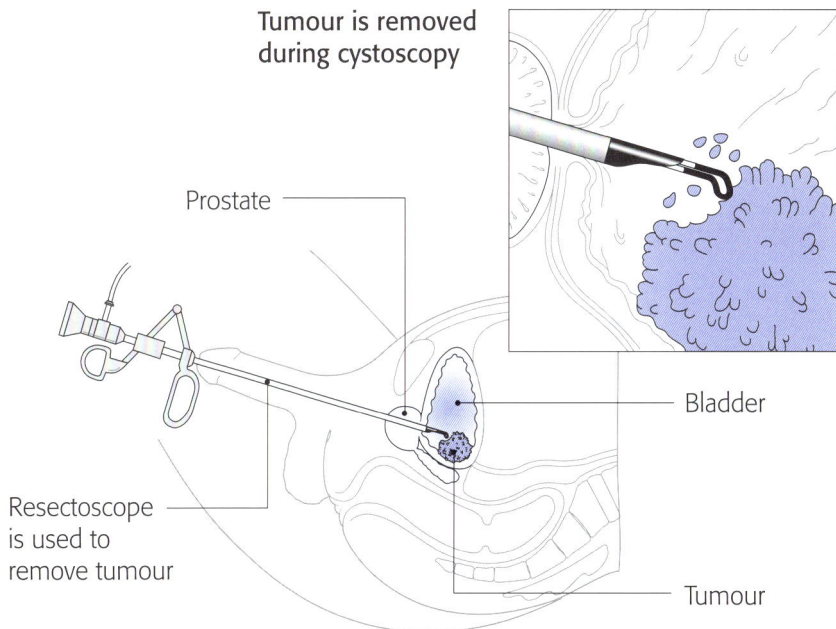

25

Tumour is removed during cystoscopy

Prostate

Resectoscope is used to remove tumour

Bladder

Tumour

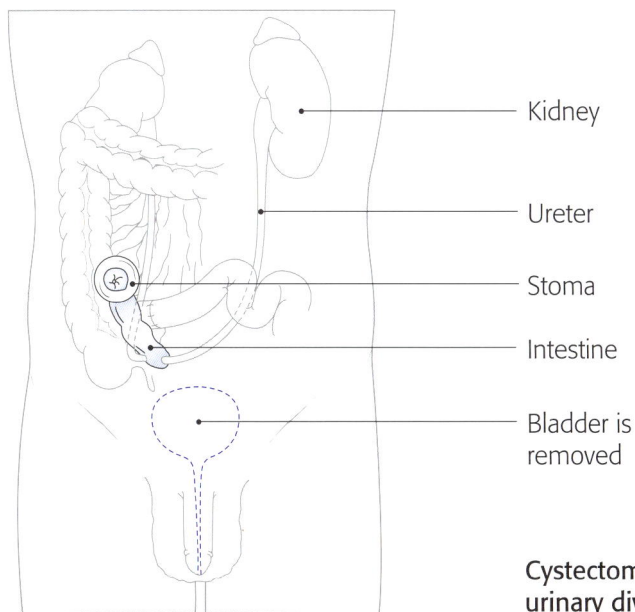

Kidney

Ureter

Stoma

Intestine

Bladder is removed

Cystectomy and urinary diversion

Cystitis

- Cystitis is inflammation of the bladder caused by infection. Patients with cystitis often feel a burning sensation when they pass urine, and need to go to the toilet more often than usual. It may also cause discomfort in the lower abdomen. The urine may be cloudy, have a strong smell and be bloodstained.

- Cystitis is more common in women because the urethra is short, making it easier for bacteria to reach the bladder. In men, the urethra is longer and cystitis is usually caused by obstruction.

- In both men and women, any disorder that obstructs the flow of urine or leads to incomplete emptying of the bladder can increase the risk of cystitis. Such disorders include kidney and bladder stones, and narrowing of the urethra. The most common cause of obstruction in men is enlargement of the prostate gland.

- You will be asked to provide a fresh sample of urine in a special, sterile container. This will be sent to the laboratory to find out which bacteria caused the infection. Collect the sample when you are in the middle of urinating.

- Cystitis is usually treated with a course of antibiotics. Other measures that may help to prevent further attacks of cystitis include drinking plenty of fluids, especially cranberry juice, and taking showers rather than baths.

- An ultrasound scan of the kidneys and bladder may be necessary for some patients.

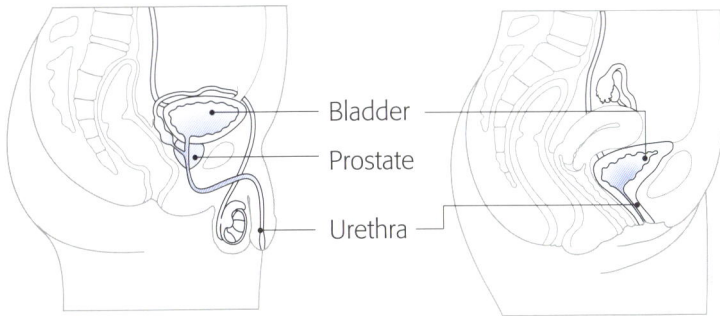

26

The urethra is longer in men than in women

- Bladder
- Prostate
- Urethra

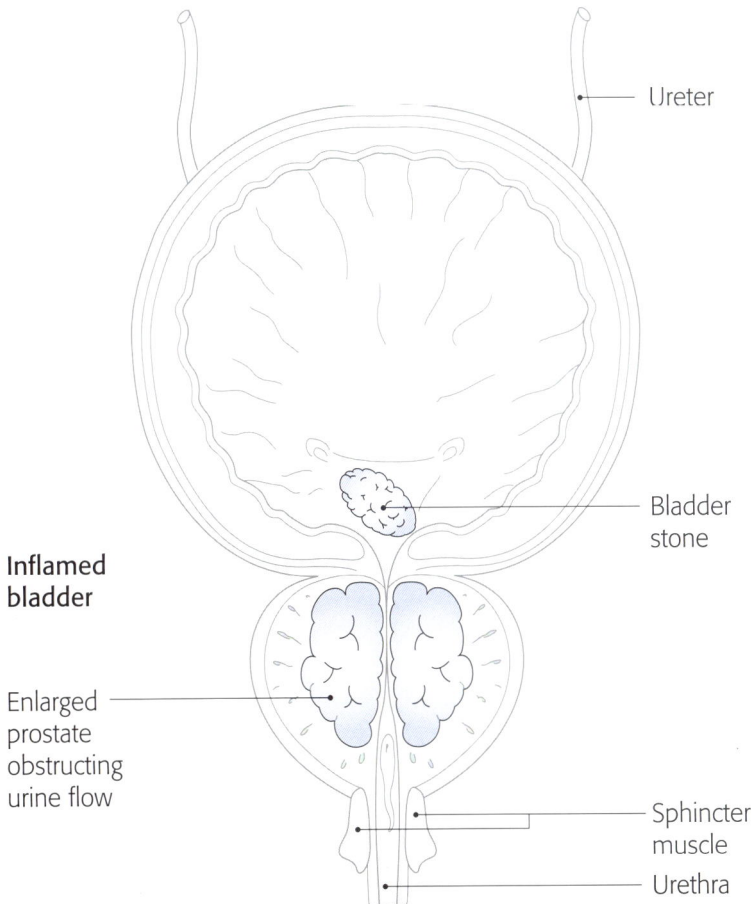

- Ureter
- Bladder stone
- Sphincter muscle
- Urethra

Inflamed bladder

Enlarged prostate obstructing urine flow

Chronic interstitial cystitis

- Some people pass urine frequently. This may be due to a disease that can be diagnosed using urodynamic tests. However, if these tests are negative, the patients are said to have a 'hypersensitive bladder'.

- In some cases, increasing the volume of fluid that the bladder can hold may help to relieve the symptoms. This involves carrying out a procedure called cystodistension under a general anaesthetic. The bladder is stretched by filling it with water under pressure, rather like blowing up a balloon.

- Occasionally, the bladder lining appears to be inflamed, but no infection can be found. This is called interstitial cystitis. It is not known what causes interstitial cystitis, but it may be an inherited condition. It is much more common in women than in men, and in some cases can cause a lot of pain.

- If the symptoms of interstitial cystitis are not relieved by stretching the bladder, washing the bladder out with a special solution of drugs may help. This involves inserting a catheter up the urethra into the bladder. The solution is then put into the bladder through the catheter and left there for half an hour. You may feel some discomfort, but a local anaesthetic will be used to ease this.

- Drug treatment with pentosan polysulfate sodium, cimetidine, amitriptyline or hydroxyzine may also help to improve the symptoms of interstitial cystitis.

27

Cystodistension

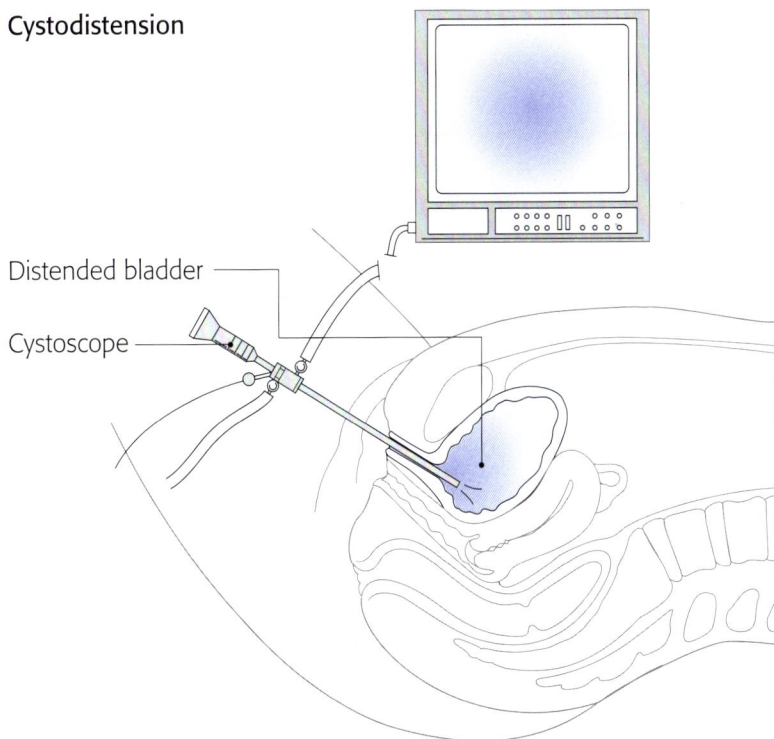

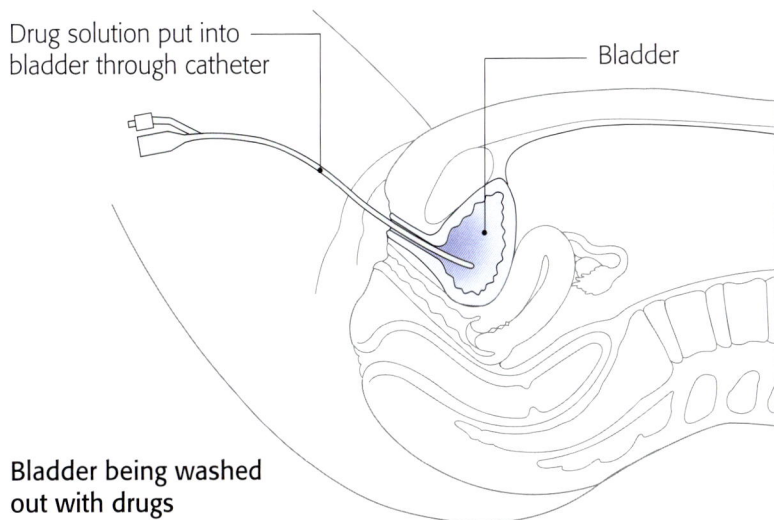

Distended bladder

Cystoscope

Drug solution put into
bladder through catheter

Bladder

**Bladder being washed
out with drugs**

Diverticula and stones

- If the flow of urine from the bladder has been obstructed for a long time, as happens in men with an enlarged prostate gland, the wall of the bladder becomes stretched. Eventually, small pouches called diverticula form in weak areas of the wall. The urine that collects in these pouches can become infected.

- The diverticula may shrink if the obstruction to the flow of urine can be treated by surgery. However, another operation is sometimes needed to remove the diverticula.

- Obstruction of the flow of urine can also lead to the formation of stones. These stones can accumulate in the bladder. They irritate the bladder and cause further obstruction. In most cases, the stones can be seen on an X-ray.

- Most bladder stones can be removed during a procedure called a cystoscopy. Small stones can be removed whole, while larger stones can be broken up into fragments with a special instrument. The fragments are washed out of the bladder with water or a dilute solution of salt.

- Sometimes it may be necessary to remove a stone surgically through an incision in the lower abdomen.

- It is best to treat the obstruction of the flow of urine to prevent further stones from developing.

28

Diverticula

Bladder stone

Bladder

Prostate

Enlarged prostate

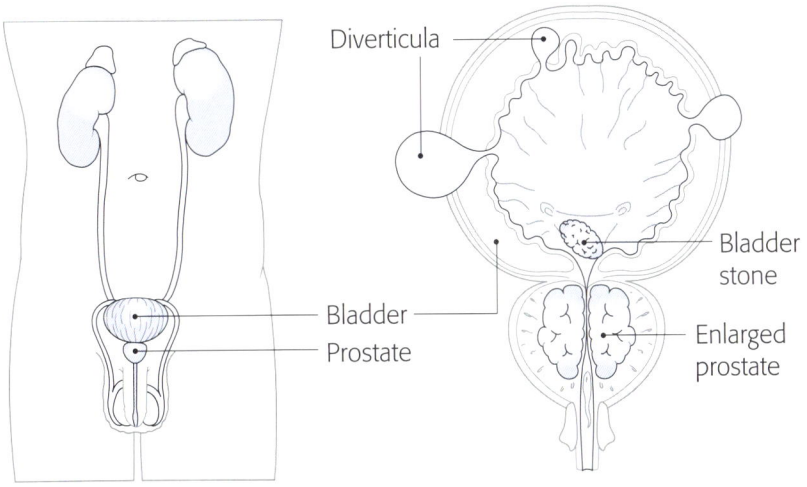

Removal of bladder stones

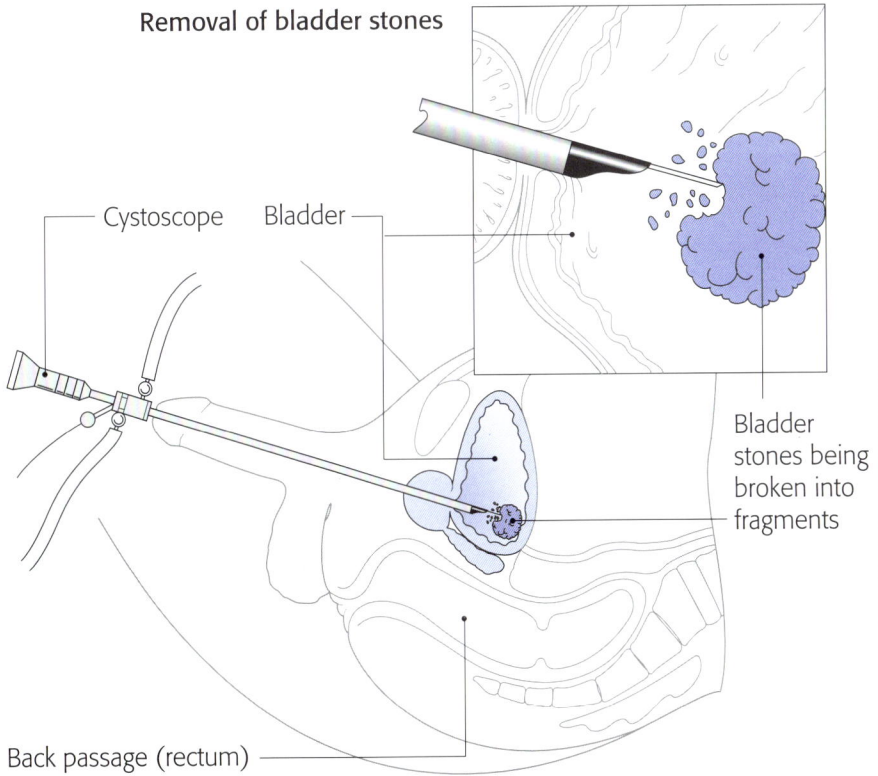

Cystoscope

Bladder

Bladder stones being broken into fragments

Back passage (rectum)

Hypocontractile bladder

- Some patients lose the ability to contract their bladder when passing urine. This is called bladder hypocontractility.

- Patients with bladder hypocontractility may take a long time to pass urine, pass small volumes frequently and be unable to empty the bladder completely. This increases the risk of urinary tract infection, which may recur frequently and may affect the kidneys. These infections can often be prevented by taking a low dose of antibiotics every day.

- Treatment with drugs called cholinergic agonists, such as carbachol or bethanechol, may be helpful when the problem is not too severe. These drugs make the bladder contractions stronger during urination. However, drugs do not usually work in more severe cases or over a long period of time.

- Patients with severe problems caused by bladder hypocontractility may need to learn a technique called intermittent clean self-catheterization, which will enable them to empty their bladder completely. This usually has to be carried out once or twice a day.

- In some cases, an operation called a urinary diversion may become necessary. This involves bypassing the bladder, and making an opening in the abdominal wall for the urine to drain through into a bag.

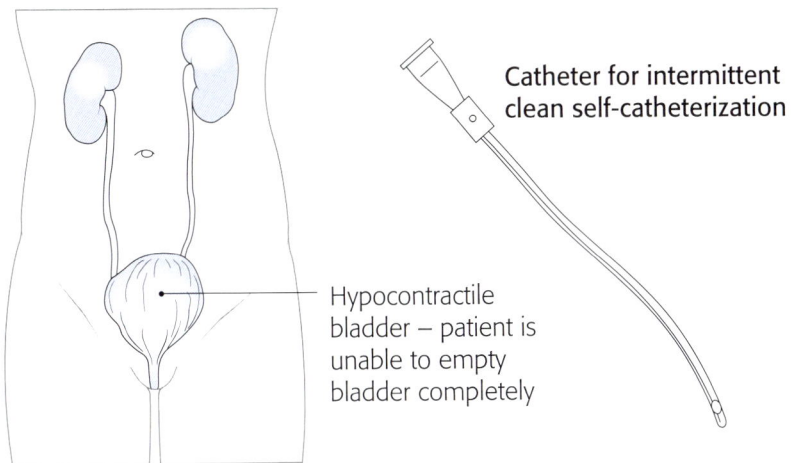

29

Catheter for intermittent clean self-catheterization

Hypocontractile bladder – patient is unable to empty bladder completely

Urinary diversion

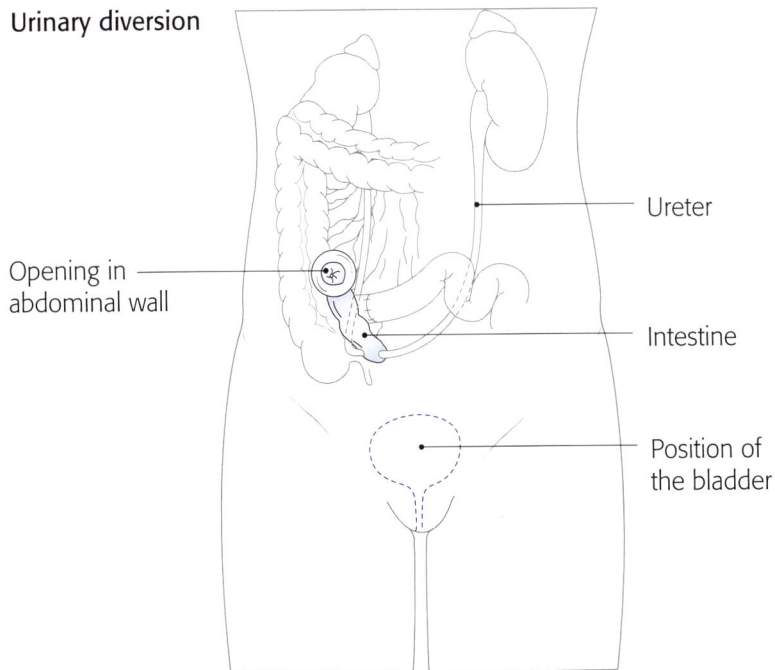

Opening in abdominal wall

Ureter

Intestine

Position of the bladder

Neuropathic bladder

- Long-term, nervous diseases that affect the spinal cord and some that affect the brain may cause bladder problems. These bladder problems can usually be treated.

- In most patients with spina bifida, the bladder muscle is overactive and contracts when it should not. The urethral sphincter may also be overactive. The urethral sphincter comprises the ring of muscle around the urethra.

- When the urethral sphincter is overactive, the bladder is prevented from emptying. These problems can lead to incontinence, the formation of stones and, if untreated, can eventually lead to kidney failure.

- The bladder problems caused by damage to the spinal cord as a result of injuries or road traffic accidents will depend on where the cord has been damaged. Soon after the injury, the bladder muscle will often not contract to empty the urine, but later becomes overactive.

- The bladder may also be affected in patients with stroke, multiple sclerosis and Parkinson's disease. Patients often need to go to the toilet more often and more urgently.

- Patients may also suffer from urge incontinence, which means that they have a strong desire to pass urine and then suddenly do so without meaning to. The urethral sphincter may also be affected, particularly in patients with Parkinson's disease, and this may make it difficult to pass urine.

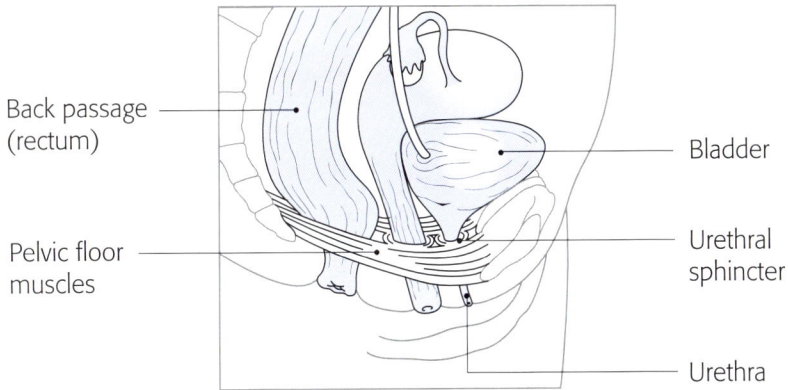

30

Back passage (rectum)

Pelvic floor muscles

Bladder

Urethral sphincter

Urethra

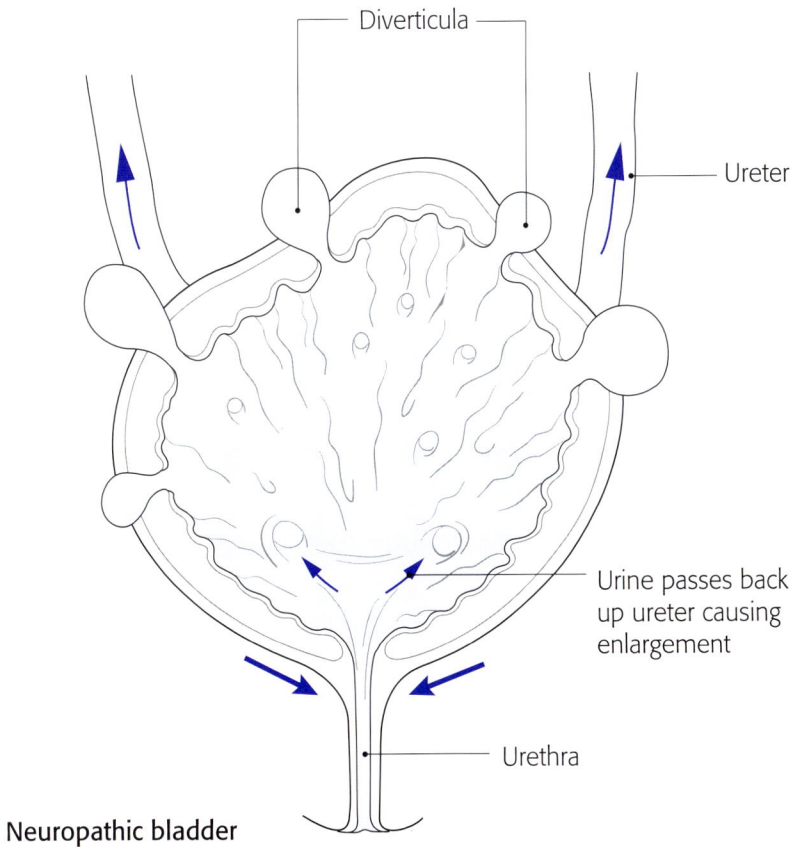

Diverticula

Ureter

Urine passes back up ureter causing enlargement

Urethra

Neuropathic bladder

Neuropathic bladder – treatment

- In neurological disease, the muscle of the bladder may be overactive. The urethral sphincter may not relax or may contract when passing urine.

- Symptoms caused by the overactivity of the bladder muscle can be treated with drugs, such as oxybutynin.

- A permanent urethral catheter will usually control the incontinence, but may cause discomfort, repeated urinary tract infections and/or become encrusted with salts found in the urine. Replacing the catheter every 3 months can help to avoid some of these problems.

- A permanent suprapubic catheter is more comfortable than a urethral catheter, especially for men. It is inserted under a local, spinal or general anaesthetic and will need to be changed about every 3 months. Patients do not usually need an anaesthetic when the catheter is changed. However, for this type of catheter to work successfully, some patients will require another operation to close the bladder neck.

- Patients with symptoms caused by problems with the bladder sphincter may need to carry out intermittent clean self-catheterization up to six times a day. This technique will enable them to empty their bladder completely.

- In some patients, urine can be diverted to an artificial opening that is made in the abdominal wall.

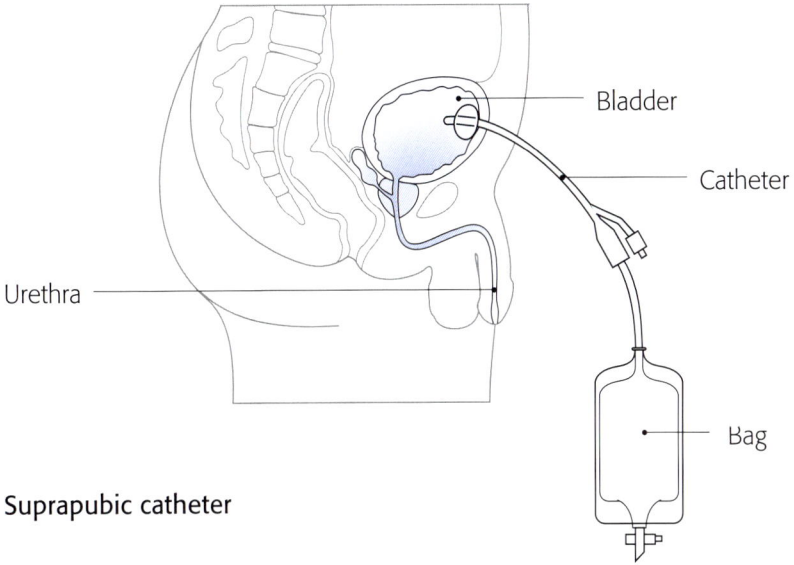

31

Bladder

Catheter

Urethra

Bag

Suprapubic catheter

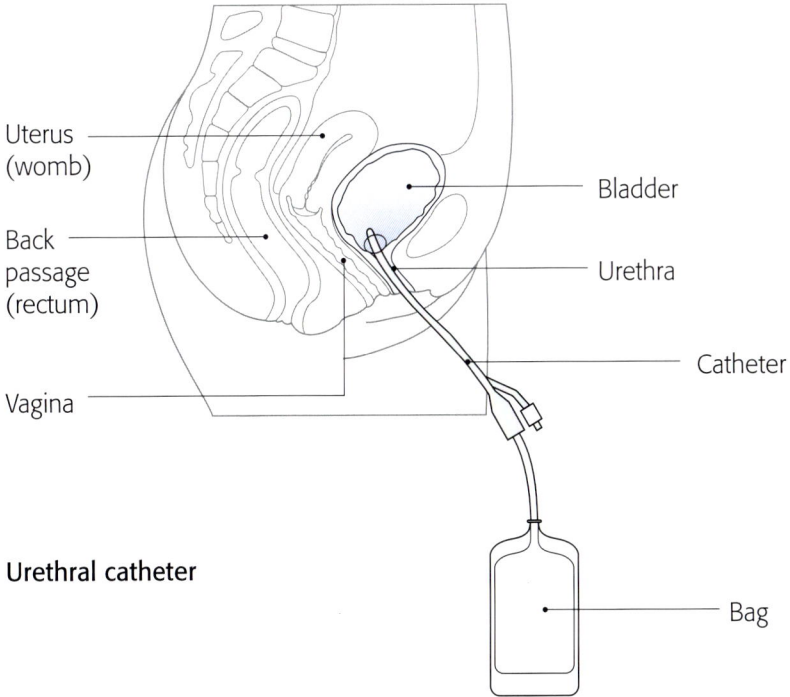

Uterus
(womb)

Back
passage
(rectum)

Vagina

Bladder

Urethra

Catheter

Bag

Urethral catheter

Urinary fistulas

- An abnormal connection can form between the bladder and other organs in the pelvis, particularly the lower bowel and the vagina. These connections are called urinary fistulas, which can lead to leakage of urine and repeated urinary tract infections.

- A vesico-vaginal fistula can lead to urine being passed through the vagina. If a colo-vesical fistula is present, stools and gas may be passed through the urethra.

- The most common cause of vesico-vaginal fistulas is damage to the bladder or ureters during surgery in the pelvic area. Colo-vesical fistulas are most commonly caused by diverticular disease, colon cancer, Crohn's disease or bladder cancer.

- A number of tests can be carried out to show the presence of a colo-vesical fistula. These include cystoscopy, cystography, sigmoidoscopy or barium enema.

- If a vesico-vaginal fistula is thought to be present, a three-swab test will be carried out. This involves putting three swabs into the vagina and a special dye into the bladder through a catheter. The swabs are then removed from the vagina.

- If the middle and innermost swabs are coloured with the dye, then a vesico-vaginal fistula is present. Other tests, for example, X-rays, may be necessary to make sure that no other damage has occurred.

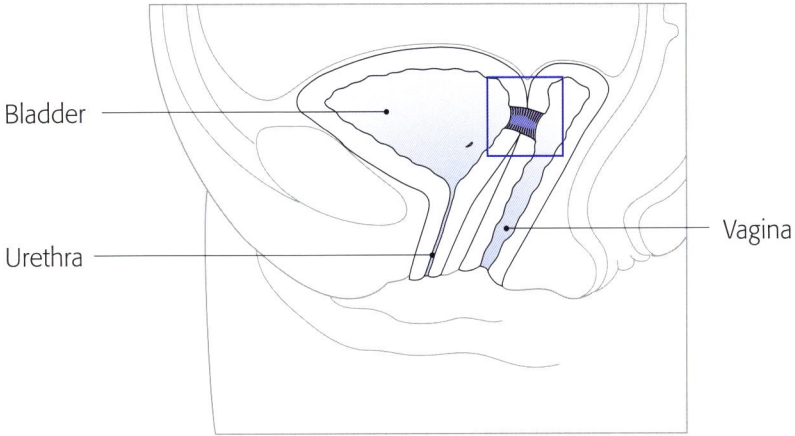

Vesico-vaginal fistula

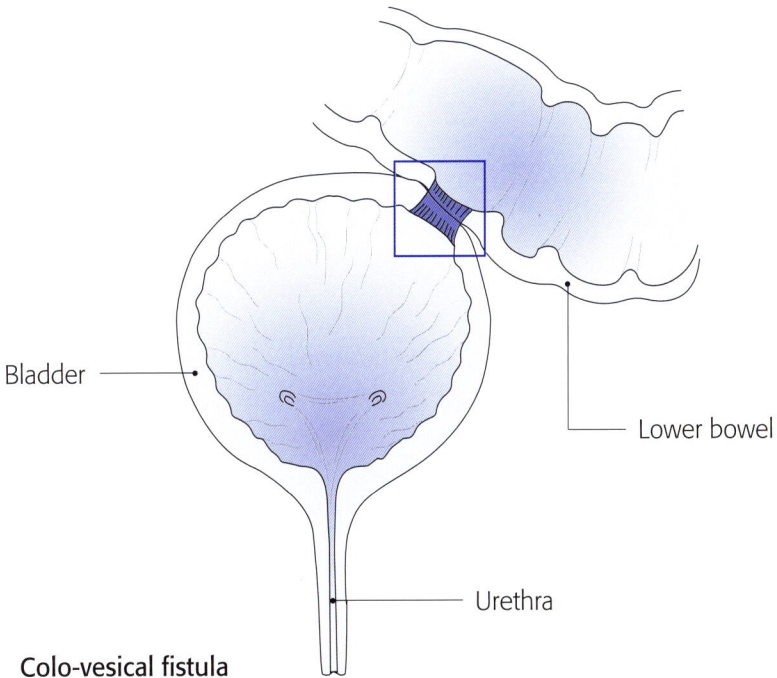

Colo-vesical fistula

Urinary fistulas – surgical treatment

- Large urinary fistulas are unlikely to heal on their own and an operation will be needed; this usually lasts 2–3 hours.

- The most successful way to repair a vesico-vaginal fistula is through a cut made in the abdomen, though repair through the vagina is sometimes possible. The tissues connecting the bladder and the vagina are removed, and the openings in the bladder and vagina closed up.

- The operation for a colo-vesical fistula is carried out through a cut made in the abdomen. However, it is important to make sure that the bowel is completely empty before the procedure. During the operation, the abnormal connection is removed and the affected section of bowel is cut away.

- Occasionally, if the bowel is obstructed in any way, it may be necessary for the surgeon to make a temporary opening in the abdomen called a colostomy. The bladder is then repaired. The temporary opening can be closed after about 3 months.

- During the operation to treat the fistula, a catheter will be passed up the urethra to drain the urine from the bladder. This will be left in place to allow the tissues to heal and will usually be removed after about 1 week. A cystogram will then be carried out. This involves taking X-rays of your bladder to ensure that the operation has been successful.

- The average hospital stay is variable, but you will feel fit and well again after about 8 weeks.

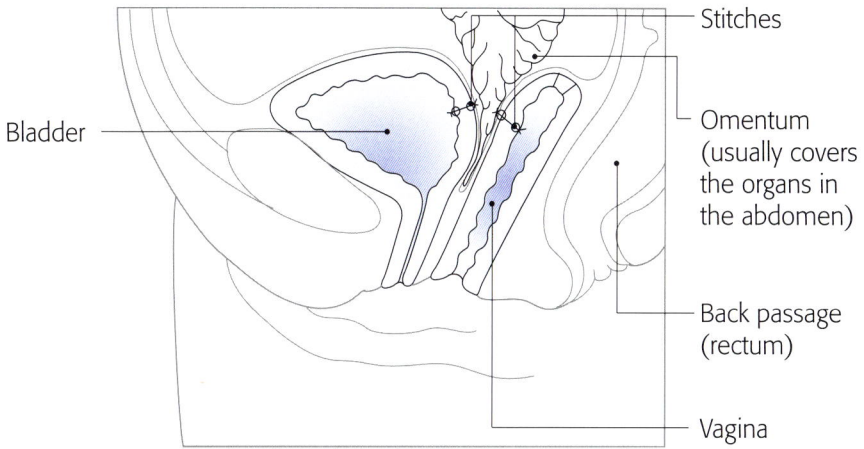

Vesico-vaginal fistula
after treatment

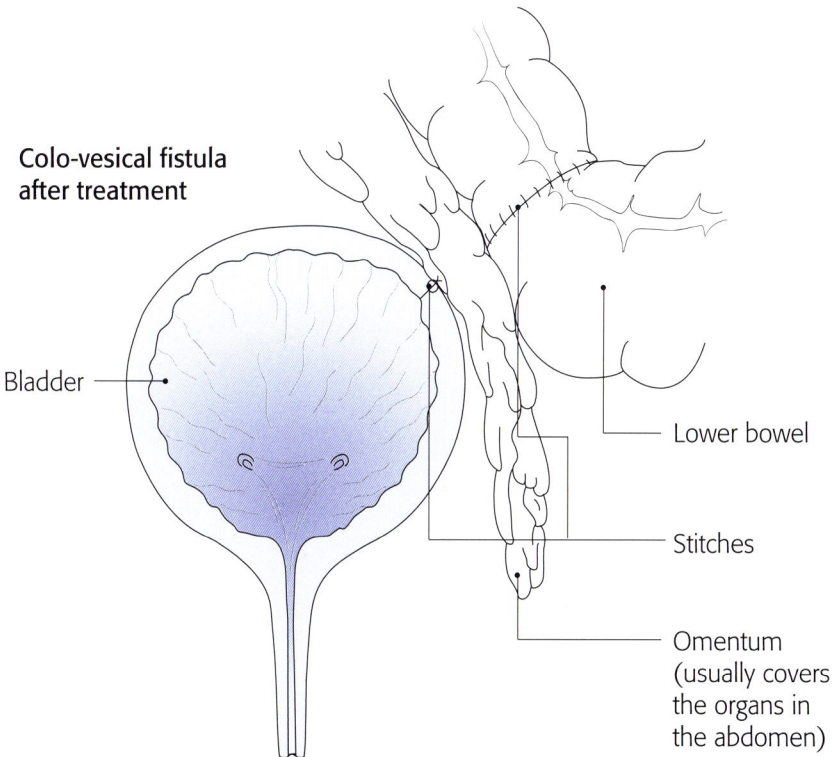

Colo-vesical fistula
after treatment

Mail Order

This *Patient Pictures* book is one of a
rapidly growing series.

Current *Patient Pictures* titles:

- *Cardiology*
- *Fertility*
- *Gastroenterology*
- *Gynaecology (2nd edition)*
- *HIV medicine*
- *Prostatic diseases and treatments*
- *Respiratory diseases*
- *Rheumatology (2nd edition)*
- *Urological surgery*

For an order form or an up-to-date
list of *Health Press* titles, simply
phone or fax:

Phone +44 (0)1235 523233
Fax +44 (0)1235 523238